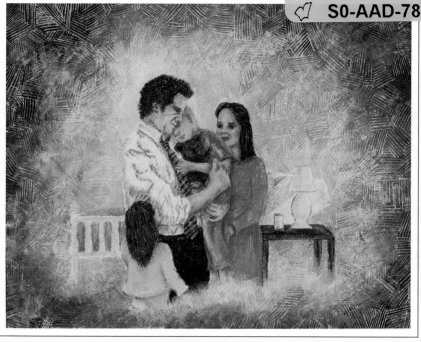

Loss

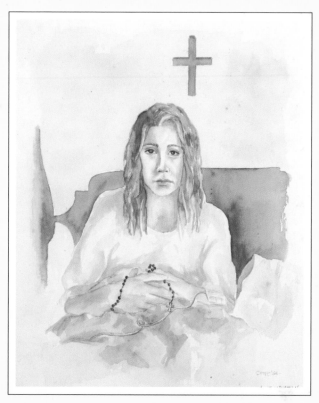

Awaiting the Comforter

Suffering

About the Artist

Connie Brill is a graphic illustrator and painter who resides in Northern California. She has worked with Dr. Betty Ferrell and colleagues at the City of Hope to illustrate the messages from patients and families regarding pain, quality of life, and suffering. For the past ten years, Connie has worked with various corporations and individuals to create diverse graphic illustrations for numerous projects.

Suffering

BETTY ROLLING FERRELL, PhD, RN, FAAN

*City of Hope National Medical Center
Duarte, California*

Jones and Bartlett Publishers

Sudbury, Massachusetts

Boston   London   Singapore

Editorial, Sales, and Customer Service Offices
Jones and Bartlett Publishers
40 Tall Pine Drive
Sudbury, MA 01776
1-508-443-5000
1-800-832-0034

Jones and Bartlett Publishers International
7 Melrose Terrace
London W6 7RL
England

Library of Congress Cataloging-in-Publication Data

Suffering / [edited by] Betty Rolling Ferrell.
   p.   cm.
   Includes bibliographical references and index.
   ISBN 0-86720-723-X
   1. Sick—Psychology. 2. Suffering. 3. Pain. 4. Stress
(Psychology) I. Ferrell, Betty.
   [DNLM: 1. Stress, Psychological. 2. Pain—psychology.
3. Disease—psychology. 4. Professional-Patient Relations. WM 172
S9448 1996]
R726.5.S825   1996
155.9—dc20
DNLM/DLC
for Library of Congress   95-544
                                       CIP

Credits
Acquisitions Editor: Jan Wall
Manufacturing Buyer: Dana L. Cerrito
Design: Pat Torelli, Solar Script, Inc.
Editorial Production Service: Solar Script, Inc.
Illustrations: Asterisk Group, Inc.
Typesetting: Kachina Typesetting, Inc.
Cover Design: Hannus Design Associates
Printing and Binding: Braun-Brumfield, Inc.
Cover Printing: Henry N. Sawyer Co., Inc.
Cover Artist: Connie Breel

Printed in the United States of America

99 98 97 96 95   10 9 8 7 6 5 4 3 2 1

Contents

Foreword

READING THE PROFESSIONAL LITERATURE, one often gets an impression that *pain* and *suffering* are used as synonymous terms. The articles in this book provide cogent reminders that such is not the case. Pain as response to disease or injury is not the same as that sense of disruption and fractured identity experienced as suffering. Although pain can contribute to suffering, suffering as lived experience occurs when the meaning of a person's life situation has been ruptured by one or more salient changes that bring a diminished sense of what it means to be human.

The dimensions of lived experience that can be precursors to suffering are (a) bodily changes that interfere with one's physical or mental access to the world; (b) interferences with interpersonal relationships and connections to other people; (c) discrepancies between one's ideals and principles and one's actions, resulting in a loss of personal integrity; and (d) disconnection between identified purpose in living and a sense of belonging to an ordered world or being part of a coherent belief system (2).

Serious illness contributes to suffering because it impinges to a greater or lesser degree on all of these dimensions that give meaning to human existence. Powerful symbols of death, disability, and unrelenting pain, diseases such as cancer and AIDS create situations that foster alienation and anguish in patients, fear and exhaustion in family members, helplessness and loss of control in health care providers.

For each person, suffering is a private experience. It derives from a unique biographical journey through time in interaction with a current life situation that threatens some aspect of personal identity. Yet the meanings ascribed to suffering and the behaviors used to express suffering to others are learned through interpersonal transactions and social activities in particular cultural contexts that Kleinman (1) calls local moral worlds. In other words, suffering occurs as part of an ongoing flow of interpersonal engagements in which participants are guided in their relationships by deep aspirations and goals, perceived threats, and beliefs about ultimate meanings such as the nature of life and death and the position of humans in the universe.

Through interpersonal experiences in the context of their everyday lives, people are introduced to religious and other cultural meanings of suffering. They learn to associate cultural meanings of suffering. They learn to associate anguish and distress, markers of suffering, with certain types of events, such as bereavement after the loss of a loved one and catastrophic accidents in which survivors are overwhelmed by mass destruction, death, and human misery. Through experiences in families and neighborhoods they learn ways of responding to distress in other people; they learn ways of protecting themselves from being engulfed in feelings of despair in response to perceived miseries in others.

Although suffering is assumed to be a universal human experience, across cultures ways of responding to suffering in oneself and in others vary considerably. Differences in perceptions, expectations, and overt behaviors can lead to conflicts and misunderstandings when people from different cultural backgrounds come together in a context of suffering. Misunderstandings and conflicting images of suffering make it easy to isolate those who are different or to treat them in dehumanizing ways through use of stereotypes and denigrating labels. In any multicultural society, such as the United States, these negative communication patterns are not uncommon.

Contacts with the health care system for those with serious illness can lead to depersonalizing experiences for many. The culture of health care is built around medically centered diagnosis and treatment activities—not to the amelioration of suffering in patients and families. The discomfort and distress associated with disease processes and the uncertainties of illness can be heightened by new experiences with tests and treatments that hurt, frequent contacts with many different providers, and difficulties in obtaining information about the current situation and the future.

Workers in health care generally are focused on controlling symptoms, implementing medical treatments, monitoring signs of recovery or movement into a chronic or terminal state of disease. Planning with patients often centers on the illness and its management, and patients may or may not feel free to share with nurses, physicians, or social workers their real concerns and fears. Yet some patients likely are struggling with feelings of loss, worries about becoming a burden on others, fears of dying abandoned by family and friends. Opportunities to share such concerns and fears with an understanding and supportive provider can serve to counterbalance the loneliness of suffering and to promote integrity of the person.

Unlike pain, which is a symptom to be managed, suffering is an all-encompassing experience of the person that must be endured or lived through alone. Yet suffering may be more bearable in the presence of concerned others who acknowledge its existence and function as human connections during a time of personal disruption and inner struggle to find meaning. Special opportunities exist for physicians and nurses to provide that human connection in their encounters with suffering patients, family members, and colleagues. To do so requires a willingness to enter into a human-to-human engagement that is not prescribed in written guidelines and protocols and that can trigger personal feelings of discomfort and loss of control.

The contributors to this collection of essays help to inform us about the many ways by which pain and illness can interfere with the ongoing life experience of being human. Some remind us of the special vulnerabilities of infants and children, the poignant experiences of persons with AIDS, the impact of living with cancer on the daily lives of patients and families, the meaning of survivorship. Some explore relationships between theoretical perspectives on pain and suffering and empirical observations about patients and families. Others consider the meaning of suffering from the professional perspectives of medicine, theology, and nursing. Together these essays are reminders of just how much pain and suffering are part and parcel of the work world of health care. They also are reminders that professional providers have many opportunities to make a difference in the lives of suffering people, not only by attending to the relief of pain and other distressing symptoms but also by listening to their underlying concerns and being present with them during moments of despair. Caregiving may well be an art form that brings together professional expertise and know-how with a sense of when a situation calls for human-to-human communication and concern more so than expert knowledge and skill.

REFERENCES

1. Kleinman, A. (1992). Local worlds of suffering: An interpersonal focus for ethnographies of illness experience. *Qualitative Health Research, 2,* 127–134.
2. Rawlinson, M. C. (1986). The sense of suffering. *The Journal of Medicine and Philosophy, 11,* 39–62.

Jeanne Quint Benoliel
Professor Emeritus University of Washington

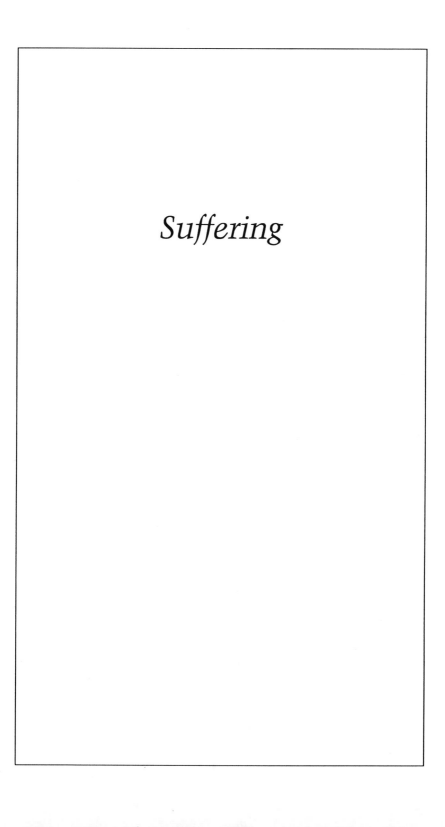

Suffering

Part One

The Experience of Suffering

Sharing a Final Chapter

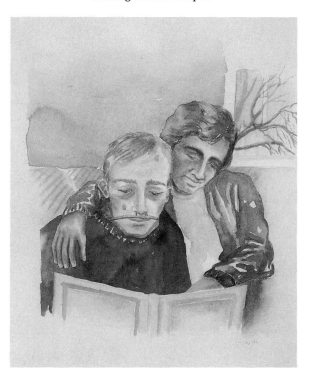

Chapter 1

An Understanding of Suffering Grounded in Clinical Practice and Research

David L. Kahn, PhD, RN   *The University of Texas at Austin*

Richard H. Steeves, PhD, RN, FAAN   *University of Virginia*

THE TWO OF US, Kahn and Steeves, first began to work together in the 1980s, when we were graduate students at the University of Washington School of Nursing. We had both been drawn to work with Jeanne Quint Benoliel, who was renown for her work in the fields of breast cancer and death and dying. It was during an independent study with Dr. Benoliel in which we explored together the intricacies of phenomenological and hermeneutic approaches to research, an area that was new to the three of us, that we began to formulate the research interest in suffering and meaning that has dominated our scholarly careers to date.

Initially, Kahn brought with him a background in comparative religion and anthropology. Steeves, on the other hand, had a master's degree in fine arts in creative writing and brought with him an abiding interest in the way people make meaning in their lives through the use of language. It was Jeanne Benoliel's suggestion that we study suffering, a suggestion that immediately made sense to us both. From Steeves' point of view, the experience in life that was most difficult to make sense of and thus was most important in terms of making meaning was suffering. From Kahn's point of view, suffering was a quintessential human experience that transcended the boundaries of human culture— understanding how people suffered and made meaning of their suffering would provide insight into the fundamental nature of humanness. Perhaps there are other, more powerful reasons for both of us to be drawn to the subject of suffering, but these remain deeply hidden and personal, best left for others to interpret.

Since our early study with Benoliel, over the past decade, we have begun to achieve, at least somewhat, an understanding of suffering that has relevance for nursing science and practice. We have done theoretical and conceptual work on the topic and have conducted empirical studies. Our work has been informed by what we have read in the literature and what the participants in our studies have told us. As well, we have gained valuable insight from our clinical work as hospice nurses. The remainder of this chapter will be a discussion of what we believe we now understand about the phenomenon of suffering. The presentation will take the form of a chronological account of how we moved from one avenue of thought to another, until our arrival at this point which we regard as a momentary interlude in our passage—thus, a travelogue, so to speak, written only part way through the journey.

Early Theoretical Work

Our first work in the area of suffering was based on a critical review of several bodies of literature (1). In this work, we attempted to set forth the relevance that theoretical development of suffering would have for nursing science and to, therefore, stimulate scholarly discourse in the nursing literature about suffering. At the time, most discussion of suffering in the literature was obscured by extant conceptual confusion of suffering with physical pain. Although most authors acknowledged that suffering was different from pain and other things that could cause suffering, the distinction was never elaborated very well. When it came down to discussion of actual practice and human beings, the tendency was to consider suffering as a degree of pain or some other kind of distress, instead of a distinct experience that took place on the level of the whole person. This is a problem that Cassell noted as well in the medical literature in his classic article about suffering (2).

Based on our literature review, we advanced a theoretical definition of suffering as an individual's experience of threat to self, a meaning given to events such as pain or loss. As Spross observed, a contribution of this definition was the "recognition that suffering is not necessarily a perception or sensation but an *evaluation* of the significance or meaning of pain" as well as other potential suffering-inducing experiences (3, p. 72). The critical components for us then, and still in any definition of suffering, are the notion of whole person or self, of an event or loss that threatens that self, and that the level of this interaction is of personal experience. The prime distinction is that it is the relationship between the event and the self that determines suffering rather than any inherent characteristics of the event itself. Suffering then must be viewed as a lived experience that is unique to each person. Other recent definitions of suffering have acknowledged the subjective nature of suffering (4), (5), (6), (7).

Another line of thinking that we followed in our early work arose out of our clinical practice. In another paper, we recounted several stories that came from our practices or from colleagues in hospice nursing (8). These stories exemplified what we called "experiences of meaning." In this paper we began to explore the relationship between suffering and meaning.

What we proposed was that suffering was a threat not only to self but to a sense of meaning in life. We eventually realized that these are one and the same. That is, the self is a set of meanings or understandings of the world and one's place in the world. A threat to the self is a disruption in the understanding of what the world is about, and this disruption is suffering.

In the narratives we explored about hospice patients and their families, we noticed that the people in them expressed the disruption of their understanding of their world by raising questions—"Why does this have to happen to me?", "Why must I die now?", or "Why must I be left alone in the world?" The patients and family members wondered about how they could bear the loss of dying or the loss of their loved one. They no longer understood the existential situation of their lives and how they could continue to live in face of this lack of understanding. This lack of understanding was often expressed in terms of loss of self or part of self.

In the face of this suffering, the patients and family members in the narratives we collected had "experiences of meaning." These were discrete moments of transcendence in which they were able to step outside of their specific circumstances, their existential situations, and understand life in terms of larger patterns of meaningfulness. Examples included a person who spoke of transcending her suffering in her garden as she pruned her roses and a man who lost his suffering and regained his self for a moment in listening to music from his youth.

These narratives were collected from a small subset of hospice patients. We came to see that these discrete and dramatic experiences of meaning were only one way in which suffering could be ameliorated, and that the environmental conditions under which such experiences occurred were unpredictable. Our attention was drawn to the way conditions in the environment potentially affected the individual's experience of suffering, especially conditions related to social interaction.

The Language of Nursing Study

Our next work in the area of suffering grew out of our concern with social interaction and suffering. Specifically, we became interested in the relationships and interactions between people experiencing suffering and those who care for them. In a qualitative study, we looked at the language a group of nurses used to describe the suffering and coping of patients and their own caring for them, as well as collected stories that epitomized suffering, caring, and coping for these nurses. The formal reports of these findings, as well as a full description of the methods of data collection and analysis, are in the nursing literature; a complete reiteration of these findings is beyond the scope of this chapter (9), (10), (11).

However, two areas from this study bear some discussion here in the impact they had on how we thought about suffering. First, we developed a simple interactional model that described the relationship of suffering with caring and coping as illustrated in Figure 1–1. This model can be viewed as the clinical context of suffering.

In this model, suffering is represented as the apex of a triangle with caring and coping at the base. The assumption is that suffering is a central experience that motivates and guides the responses of coping and caring. Caring is a response of other persons, including nurses, to the sufferer. Coping, on the other side of the triangle, is the person's own response to his or her suffering. The caring efforts of others and the coping efforts of self continually respond and modify each other. We will return to this model in a more developed form at the end of this chapter.

The second area of this study that we will discuss here involves our analysis of the stories nurses told us about the suffering of patients and families they encountered in their clinical practices (10). The clustering of themes about suffering in the nurses' stories could be interpreted as a progression of the nurses' own understanding of the suffering they encountered in their clinical practices. Specifically, the nurses tended to first conceive of suffering as a patient condition. This

FIGURE 1–1

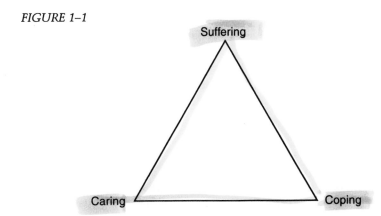

was in line with the "medical model" view of illness reducible to conditions and treatments that dominated the settings in which they had practiced. Yet, immediately this understanding of suffering was not satisfying for the nurses because ways in which suffering deviated from the medical model world view were readily apparent to them, as were numerous ways in which individuals' suffering were not open to detached, objective scrutiny.

The next understanding of suffering the nurses in this study had was of suffering as a human experience. The nurses were well aware of the complexity of suffering and the uniqueness of suffering as experienced by different individuals. Their poignant narratives were thick, rich descriptions of memorable patients and family members, filled with tragedy, irony, and considerable courage.

The understanding of suffering as a human experience did not completely satisfy the nurses in this study either. They still found the subject troubling and laden with emotion. Their final understanding of suffering was a personal one. The nurses recognized their emotions in reaction to the suffering encountered on a daily basis in clinical practice and their feelings of helplessness in the face of this reality. For some of the nurses, it was a short, difficult step from this realization to the personalization of suffering. The suffering became their own.

In order to understand this interpretation of our data, we turned to Marris's theory of meaning structures and human adaptability (12). Marris theorized that humans respond to new experiences by depending on familiar, always established cognitive-emotional structures. These structures enable the person to give a meaning to the new experience that maintains a sense of continuity with previous experience. In this regard, the initial understanding of suffering by the nurses in terms of the familiar and established medical model makes sense.

However, their experiences with individual patients caused them to discredit the assumptions of that familiar structure and revise and reformulate new structures of meaning. According to Marris, in order to reestablish the sense of continuity in the face of the loss of familiar assumptions requires a process of bereavement in which a new understanding of the situation is attained and emotional responses worked through (12).

In applying Marris's theory to our analysis, a new insight into and understanding of suffering emerged. The experience of suffering could be viewed as the gap or abyss that opens when one meaning structure has been challenged or destroyed and a new one has not been formed. The gap is the time when things that happen to a person are no longer explainable by any system of making sense of things, of why things happen. Suffering then could be defined not as a meaning given to events that threaten personal identity but as meaninglessness caused by that very threat.

Two Studies of Suffering and Meaning in Different Clinical Populations

Our next research studies were individual projects, although conceived in collaboration to complement each other. In both studies we attempted to investigate patterns of suffering and meaning within different groups of individuals experiencing the same potentially threatening events, and thus exposed to the possibility of suffering. Steeves took a prospective approach, choosing to describe the experiences of six young men who underwent allogenic bone marrow transplantation for treatment of leukemia (13). In contrast, Kahn's approach was an investigation of the experiences of a group of aged residents of a nursing home for Jewish elders (14).

The Bone Marrow Transplant Study

At the cancer center in which Steeves' study was conducted, the protocol for bone marrow transplants (BMT) was 100 days long, from the point of infusion of the new bone marrow until patients could go home to their own community. Steeves recruited his participants two to three weeks before the actual transplantation and followed them through all stages of BMT: the outpatient data gathering stage; the inpatient conditioning that consisted of high doses of total body irradiation coupled with chemotherapy; the stage of severe stomatitis during which they could not speak; the inevitable complications such as infections, veno occlusive disease, and graft versus host disease; and finally their slow recovery or decline toward death. Steeves spent time with each participant almost every day, taperecording conversations and taking field notes. Over time, he established rapport with the participants' extended families as well. At the end of the study, two participants were disease-free and well enough to return home. The other four participants had died.

The study provided both methodological and substantive insights in our exploration of suffering. Methodologically, there were two problems. First, a tremendous amount of data were gathered, and it was necessary to find a method to reduce the data enough to make specific points without losing the essence of the experience from the participants' perspective. Second, in a prospective study in which the participants are recruited on the basis of the expectation that they may experience some suffering (but which has not yet started) it is difficult to ask them about their suffering as they endure difficult experiences without changing the way the participants think about those experiences.

The first problem was solved using a technique that has become increasingly important in our ongoing research. Instead of grouping all the data across participants and searching for themes and patterns, Steeves decided to construct the story of each participant. With the advantage of knowing how each story ended, crucial aspects of each day for each participant were selected and arranged in chronological order. The end product was a narrative account of the experience of each participant containing the details necessary to move the narrative forward and make it coherent.

The second problem was solved through a strategy of asking different questions of the participants and of the data. That is, the participants were asked to talk about what was happening to them. They were asked to describe what they were going through and how they felt about it. Later, as the data were reduced and the narrative for each participant constructed, Steeves asked, "What do these stories tell about the nature of suffering?"

The findings of the BMT study included a description of the themes that characterized suffering for these men and a description of their activities aimed at alleviating or coping with their suffering. The themes that characterized suffering for these BMT patients were (a) the loss of time, causing them to believe their futures and their lives were no longer their own, (b) a fundamental change in their social relationships, and (c) a change in their relationship with their own bodies.

Time was an important theme for these men, because they were told that they had no future without the BMT and that their chances for having a future with the BMT were uncertain. They were not able to dream or plan for any future for themselves. For example, one of the participants was an 18-year-old high school senior who, before he became ill, had college plans and had even been admitted to the school he wanted. He also had a girlfriend. He felt compelled to give up both and declared that he could no longer think about them.

Because of the BMT, these six men also lost control of their present time. Instead of choosing how they would spend their time, their days had to be structured around the routine of the hospital unit and the necessities of their treatment regimen. For example, the men were told when and how they had to bathe, how often and how much they must eat, and were given a long list of the special services (e.g., respiratory and physical therapy) whose personnel would be visiting them.

The social changes the participants of this study underwent resulted from the BMT treatments and consequences. Not only were participants a long way from their homes, all having traveled to a national center for BMT, their social isolation was increased by the need for strict reverse isolation procedures. The number of their visitors was limited, and skin-to-skin touching was prohibited. Oddly enough, this isolation was accompanied by an almost total loss of privacy. The participants were often so ill or so incapacitated that they required help with the most intimate aspects of their lives including toileting and hygiene. One participant was on an experimental protocol that called for regular doses of heparin, an anticoagulant, in the hope that it would help maintain his liver function. As a result, he bled so heavily into the tissues of his hands where blood samples were drawn that he was no longer able to make a fist or grasp objects. This young bachelor resented having to be fed by his nurses and was mortified when one day—with his family out of the room—a nurse had to hold the urinal for him as he used it.

Also, during long periods of time, the men were unable to speak because of severe mouth pain related to the radiation-induced stomatitis. Accompanying the changes in the way these men were able to relate socially to others, was a strong sense of guilt because they were consuming their families' resources while no longer able to contribute the way they had. One of the participants was from Florida. His brother had given up his job there to accompany the patient to the Pacific Northwest to be his bone marrow donor and had remained to be available for platelet donations as well. This brother had found a job as a carpenter and was helping to pay for the apartment where the family lived. Two of his three school-aged children had accompanied him. One was going to the school the research center provided; the other was depending on a scholarship the local Catholic school had donated. Before the participant died in the hospital, he watched all his savings consumed so that his family could be by his side.

Usually the relationship with one's own body is transparent and not thought or talked about in everyday life until it becomes a problem for the self in some way (15), (16). The problematic nature of their bodies was obvious to the six BMT patients in this study. Most of the normal physical functions and activities, previously taken for granted, were disrupted for them. At times they were not able to sleep and at other times they were not able to stay awake. They had no appetite but were required to eat a certain number of calories a day before they could leave the hospital. The men lacked energy for most daily activities including thinking clearly. As an extreme example, one participant had the experience of feeling as though he were viewing his body from a vantage point outside himself. In the middle of the night, he woke and believed himself to be camping by a lake in the woods. He said he felt well and comfortable. "I looked over and saw some poor son-of-a-gun sitting on the bedroll next to me. He was all curled up in pain, looked yellow, and was throwing up." Of course, the participant was the only person in his strictly isolated room.

Loss of time, social role, and physical function were almost a total loss of self for the participants in the BMT study. Put another way, it was the loss of the meaning of their lives. Therefore, in response to this suffering these BMT patients struggled to find or create meaning. They used two general approaches to do so: (a) they renegotiated their social position in their new situation, and (b) they tried to construct an understanding of their experiences as a whole (17).

These BMT patients used a number of strategies to reestablish their social position. First, they became adept at understanding the power structure of the hospital unit. This enabled them to learn to use that power structure, by aligning themselves with the right people over the right issues, to regain a little of the control they lost when their sense of time was destroyed. They took back some of the choices they had about allocation of their time. The participants also redefined who they were and tried to reestablish a sense of self by an elaborate series of social comparisons with other patients who were doing better or worse than they were.

Nurses, believing both in the right of privacy for patients and that learning of the death or decline of another patient would adversely affect other patients, made a concerted effort to prevent patients from discovering how other patients on the BMT unit were doing. But their efforts were in vain. Patients always seemed to know what was happening in the other rooms on the unit. For instance, one participant followed closely the decline and death of the patient two doors away from him. He talked at length about the ways in which his disease, treatment, and course in the hospital were different from hers. A few days later, when another person on the unit was doing well enough to be discharged to home, he talked about the ways in which he was similar to that patient.

Finally, as a strategy to reestablish their social position, the participants sought and found a surprising sense of normalcy and affection in the social world of the hospital. They were able to accomplish this primarily through their relationships with nurses.

The attempt of these BMT patients to understand their experience as a whole was carried out on several levels. For example, participants used superstition to try to predict and control what would happen to them. There were lucky rooms and lucky hats and jinxes to avoid. Also, the men learned the language of "odds of success" that was the common parlance of the employees of this cancer research center. They again sought prediction and control by trying to manipulate their statistical odds.

On a deeper level that went beyond prediction and control, these participants sought to understand what they were experiencing. They developed a sense of altruism—they talked of what "medical science" was learning from them and what they would tell others who faced BMT to help them if they lived through it themselves. These men also relied heavily on religion. Like Job, they would decry their lack of understanding of why they had to suffer so much but would, at the same time, defer to the ultimate meaningfulness that God imbues in the world. Finally, two of the participants had transcendent experiences during which they experienced the meaning of being alive so directly that it could only be described as a visceral experience. They established a self that somehow transcended the suffering of their circumstances.

The Nursing Home Study

Kahn pursued an ethnographic study of a 145-bed nursing home for Jewish elderly in the Pacific Northwest (14). Data were collected over a nine-month period of participant observation. The study focused on the experiences of twenty-one residents who participated in audiotaped interviews and with whom Kahn developed significant rapport.

Interestingly, the participants glossed over their experiences of suffering related to old age and living in a nursing home through a shared metaphor of "going downhill." This metaphor, in several linguistic variations, summarized the participants' shared experiences of losses and threats to identity related to old age. Participants believed that the suffering of going downhill was a natural outcome of growing old. At the same time, the metaphor symbolically described a very complex temporal process of physical and social decline, a deconstruction of the self in terms of personal identity in old age. Going downhill, for the participants of this study, meant that the physical and social losses of old age had accumulated to the extent that the aged person's presence in the world was on a trajectory of decline. The participants in this study regarded their residencies in the nursing home as a consequence of the larger process of going downhill, not as a separate threat to personal identity or cause of suffering.

The experience of physical decline, a constriction of the social world, and a changed relationship with time comprised a three-part structure to the participants' experience of suffering or going downhill. The similarity of the overall structure of suffering to that noted in Steeves' BMT study is evident, although both studies were conducted independently and procedures were built in to prevent one analysis from influencing the other. The actual details that construct the themes from the data differed. That suggested to us that the overall structure of suffering as a human experience is grounded in universal, structural aspects of humanness. The varied content of the universal structure of suffering, the details so to speak, arise from the interaction of the specific event, here bone marrow transplantation and aging, with the individual's personal identity. This tentative and broad conclusion requires more empirical work for validation.

For these nursing home residents, physical decline was the paramount aspect of their experience. Physical decline included an accumulation of illnesses and physical problems that impaired participants' ability to function in the natural world. This experience of impaired embodiment escalated and accelerated over time. For example, one woman talked of her loss of mobility, recounting a progressive decline from canes to walker to elbow canes to wheelchair, ending with "Just recently, a few months, I got to where I couldn't turn myself in bed. Where they laid me down that's the way I got up in the morning."

The second aspect of physical decline for these participants was a fundamental experience of one's own frailty and vulnerability. For most participants, this experience was both symbolized and characterized by instances of falling.

Constriction of these participants' social worlds was due primarily to the loss of their opportunities to choose different kinds of social interactions. Participants increasingly became unable to perform formerly valued social roles and to do things that once had been intrinsic to their everyday lives. Thus, participants experienced dependency in various degrees in activities of daily self-care and mobility.

Another aspect of the constriction of the social world for these nursing home residents was that they had simply outlived many of the people who had once been important actors in their social worlds. They experienced their social environments as being dense with the death of others. In a poignant conversation, a participant recounted first the death of her husband, then of her friends and neighbors and even shopkeepers with whom she had done business for many years. Finally, she spoke of her nine brothers: "They're all gone, all those boys, little by little, little by little, little by little they died."

Finally, as part of their experience of going downhill in old age, the participants in this study noticed a change in their relationship to time. They spoke of this change as part of their suffering in two ways: loss of the present and loss of the future. The present was lost to participants in that they felt estranged from the modern world. The future was lost in that participants believed and acknowledged, realistically, that they had little future in this world as their own deaths were at hand.

An interesting finding in Kahn's nursing home study was that despite the great losses participants experienced as part of the personal decline of aging, they, with one notable exception, managed to maintain an overall sense of meaningfulness and an attitude of personal dignity in their daily lives as nursing home residents. The participants used multiple processes of meaning-making to maintain a sense of coherence and self-worth and to offset everyday threats to personal identity.

The exception to this is revealing in terms of the previous discussion of suffering and meaning. The acute suffering and despair of one participant, Minnie Schaefer [a pseudonym], were obvious to staff, residents, and all who interacted with her in the nursing home. She told everyone of her unhappiness, cried frequently, and spent hours in her bed, withdrawn but awake, curled into a fetal position. Most everyone in the nursing home avoided her as her emotional responses visibly upset them. Many members of the nursing staff found her sadness infectious in a way; as one nurse said, "The problem is she is so unhappy. I leave her room feeling there's no hope in this world."

Mrs. Schaefer attributed her suffering, her profound unhappiness, to a stroke that left her partially paralyzed and with severely impaired memory of her past life. This latter loss robbed her of the necessary elements of personal identity she needed to make any coherent meaning of her situation. Sources of meaning for the other nursing home residents in this study included a cultural stance toward suffering, personal history, family, and membership in a larger Jewish community. Mrs. Schaefer's inability to remember much about any of these things made it impossible for her to use them in a such a way as to formulate new meanings for herself that reduced her suffering.

For example, Mrs. Schaefer could not remember much about her family. She kept a picture of her husband who had died several years before her stroke, but said of her marriage, "It's hazy . . . other people here talk about things they remember. I don't remember anything." Although her son visited her every weekend, which she enjoyed, she was unable to remember any of the details of raising him. It was also a problem for her to be in "a Jewish place," as she no longer could identify with Judaism culturally or religiously. Lacking a past, she was unable to make any meaning of the present.

In a final interview, the immensity of Mrs. Schaefer's suffering and its effect on her daily life was most apparent in the following comment:

> It doesn't matter. I used to have dreams. Now I don't have any dreams. I don't sleep through the night. I just stay in bed thinking [long pause] but there is nothing to think about. I just don't like it. I would like to die. But I don't know how. Yes, [sobbing] I don't know how.

Mrs. Schaefer died in her sleep a month later.

Lay Caregivers of Persons with Cancer Study

The final study we wish to discuss in this chapter was an investigation of the experiences of 32 rural, southern, lay caregivers of persons with terminal cancer. Although the study was focused on caregiving, it has provided us with a number of new insights into the phenomenon of suffering.

The first aspect this study brought to our work was a reemphasis on our notion of the importance of narratives both in data collection and analysis. Our belief is that narratives are a reality—or at least one level of reality—that are not only accessible to the investigator of suffering as well as practitioners who deal with sufferers, but also of primary importance to the people in the lived experience of their daily lives (18).

People are not capable of living unmediated experiences. That is, as stated previously in our discussion of Marris's theory (12), we usually understand what we experience by fitting it with a preexisting meaning structure. If something does not fit into that system, we either fail to notice it—and therefore it is not an experience at all—or we become frightened and anxious because our perceptions or our meaning system has been called into question. When this conflict cannot be resolved, the self is threatened and suffering begins.

Through this study, we have come to believe that the meaning structures that Marris discussed are integrated into a larger overall system of meaning that creates the sense of continuity and coherence that, at least in Western culture, we call "the self." For each individual then, the system of meaning is embedded in a biographical narrative—the story of my life. From early in our lives, we tell ourselves and others this story, which takes on for each of us a reality that disguises its social construction. Certain stories are recognizable in given historical periods as culturally popular. Some of us are the heroes of our stories and each chapter is a struggle for success. Others of us are victims who have just managed to survive. For most of us, our lives are rich, complex narratives in which we play a number of roles.

In this study, we found that grief brought the story of the caregivers' lives to a premature end, leaving each of them without a sense of meaning. The sadness, despair, anger, and hopelessness that were part of grief were symptoms of the suffering that came from the loss of meaning that occurred when the coherent narrative of the caregivers' lives were disrupted. This was evident in that in order to alleviate their suffering and regain a sense of meaning in their lives, the caregivers in this study had to accomplish a set of tasks that were aimed at reestablishing their personal narratives in a coherent way (19), (20).

Three tasks in particular seemed essential in reestablishing meaningful narratives for the caregivers in this study. First, the caregivers repeated and relived the traumatic events of the initial diagnosis of terminal cancer and sometimes the suffering that filled the last hours of the person's life. The most useful metaphor for understanding this is that of a broken film that is caught in a loop, repeating itself over and over again. The bereaved person relives trauma because no next step or episode in life is yet apparent. The former story of life has abruptly ended, the cast of characters suddenly altered, and the last scenes are constantly repeated.

Over time, the repetition of the final trauma faded and was replaced by a review of the whole history of the bereaved person's relationship with the lost person. As the bereaved caregivers started to reform a narrative of their lives, they took memories of the past narrative and incorporated them. By reworking and reliving their memories, they were able to make the episode of their lives that fractured with the death other person part of a new narrative, one in which the death was understood as natural and reasonable and not a random event. As this happened, their suffering abated.

One example of this process was a women who lost her husband to lung cancer. When she was first interviewed, she asked rhetorically why this was happening to her, and why a good man like her husband had to suffer and die. She repeated the story of how he went to his doctor with what he thought was a cold and was told he had lung cancer. She detailed the night he began to cough up blood. That night, the hospice nurse had him admitted to the hospital where he died before she could join him. Her story was full of statements that began "If we had only. . . ." Self-doubt and guilt were thematic.

But as she continued to tell her story, it changed. When she reviewed her long marriage with this man, she explained that he worked on the railroad all week long. When he came home on weekends, he usually went drinking with his friends. She raised the children by herself, and there was rarely enough money. She also recognized that his smoking was the probable cause of his cancer, and she admitted to "nagging" him about quitting. As she developed this story of their life together, her grief abated.

The second task of grieving for these caregivers was to reknit the family that was torn apart by the death. If a family is understood not in terms of the usual social science metaphor of a system, but rather as a group of people who share in the same life stories, it is easy to understand the necessity for this task. Personal stories begin in the family. People learn who they are by participating in a family story with all its roles, power assignments, and family themes. When a member of the family dies, the story for each individual changes as does the ongoing story shared by all members.

The task of reknitting the family was approached differently by the men and women in the study. The women had a tendency to widen their families to include in more active roles relatives who had not been part of their nuclear families. For example, when the husband of a woman in her early 60's died, she discovered how difficult life was going to be for her since she had never learned to drive a car and did not know how to start a lawn mower. So, she became closer to her sister and her family, and the nieces and nephews began to teach her the skills she needed.

On the other hand, the men in the study who lost wives had a tendency to replace them. Often, this was sanctioned, and even encouraged, within cultural structures. For instance, a man in his 60's who was the head of a traditional Appalachian family had received support for most of his life from his Pentecostal Christian church. Within a year after his wife's death, his pastor began to call him on Saturday evenings to suggest that there was a widow who might need a ride to church the next morning.

Finally, the caregivers needed to work out a relationship with the lost person. As participants formed new narratives, they did not seem complete or satisfying until the person who had died had been added in some way to the cast of characters. For these participants then, the final task for restarting their own personal narrative in the midst of bereavement meant finding a new role for the person who had died. Such roles varied from person-to-person or narrative-to-narrative, but what held was that the deceased again became a presence in the bereaved person's life story.

An interesting example of this last point was a man in his early 40's whose wife died of breast cancer. He was faced with the task of raising two pre-school age daughters. He was angry with his wife for having died and leaving him with this responsibility. One night, several weeks after her death, his wife appeared to him in a dream. He said to her, "How could you leave me to raise the girls by myself?" She responded, "I will help you." "How can you do that?," he asked. She replied, "I can help you, but we will have to do it in the same body." The next morning he woke, put on one of her favorite necklaces under his shirt, and slipped two of her rings onto his little fingers.

Tenets of Suffering

Our research and theoretical work in suffering continues in a number of projects in progress. Recently, however, we were challenged to formulate our beliefs about suffering based on our work in a way that was accessible to clinicians as well as researchers and other scholars (21). To do this, we formulated a number of succinct statements about suffering that represent our best understanding of the phenomenon of suffering. For the remainder of this chapter, we will explicate these principles or tenets of suffering. The origin of these statements should be clear in the discussion above.

Suffering is a private lived experience of a whole person, unique to each individual. Each person's suffering is as unique as their life, for suffering is totally personal. In other words, an individual's suffering results from a particular and coincidental configuration of a situation, response to attempts to ameliorate that situation, and various aspects of everyday life that occur in combination with a person's unique personal and social identity.

Suffering results when the most important aspects of a person's identity are threatened or lost. Cassell made the same point when he defined suffering as a severely distressful experience associated with events that threaten the intactness of a person (2), (22). So did Jeanne Benoliel who noted that suffering was "the inner experience of losing a part of the self" (23).

Since suffering is dependent on the meaning of an event or loss for the individual, it can not be assumed present or absent in any given clinical condition. For each person, it is the relationship between a loss, a symptom, a diagnosis, or other event and their own identity that determines whether suffering is experienced. For example, in pain, it is not the pain itself that determines suffering but the meaning the pain has for the individual. The likely difference in meaning, for instance, of pain from childbirth versus pain related to a cancerous tumor is a clear example of this. Suffering is embedded within another experience (such as pain) that may or may not induce suffering in a given individual.

That some things will cause suffering in many people is obvious to clinicians. For example, a diagnosis of cancer that may be terminal, with attendant uncontrolled pain, will more often than not be interpreted by a person in a way that results in suffering. But many conditions are not as predictably certain as they may seem at first. For instance, Benedict's study of 30 adults who had undergone chemotherapy, radiation therapy, and/or surgery for primary pulmonary malignancies illustrates this point well (4). Although half her sample reported suffering very much, an interesting one-tenth reported that they were not suffering at all.

Suffering can also be viewed as an experience of lost personal meaning. It seems to us from our vantage point today, that what is common in all the suffering of patients and participants we've encountered in practice and research has been their struggle to regain personal meaning—the sense that life is not random but is coherent and is one in which their identities have continuity. This struggle to make or find meaning takes many faces. We described above instances in which meaning was found in the transcendence of suffering, in daily coping with changed conditions, in understanding their situation in a larger framework, and reworking and restarting coherent life narratives.

Possible sources of suffering are innumerable. To speak or write about sources of suffering is to acknowledge suffering's private nature, that the cause of suffering in any given individual is totally personal (24), (25). Numerous potential sources of suffering in cancer and other chronic conditions have been identified by various authors (3), (4), (26), (27), (28), (29), (30), (31), (32), (33), (34). Given the personal nature of suffering, potential sources of suffering are virtually limitless. Thus, focusing on possible sources of suffering in isolation, separated from individual patients, is not a useful strategy for clinical practice or research. Understanding the sources of suffering for any given individual, however, can lead to understanding of the behaviors, attitudes, and responses of the person who is suffering.

We recognize certain kinds of experiences as forms of suffering; we acknowledge these forms as experiences that will lead to suffering for many who experience them. It is useful to distinguish the private origin or source of an individual's experience of suffering from the public manifestation of that experience. To speak or write about a form of suffering then is to approach suffering from the public realm, that which is apparent to us as clinicians and members of a culture. For example, bereavement from the loss of a spouse to cancer is a readily recognizable form of suffering. Statements can be made about bereavement's typical trajectory, tasks, and alleviation as a form of suffering (19), (35). As Shweder noted, "suffering takes form when it becomes organized . . . and is experienced and expressed as suffering of a certain kind" (25, p. 481).

The expression of suffering is clearly more accessible to clinicians than the experience. Development of knowledge about forms of suffering would focus on such expression, described in anthropological terms as "idioms of distress" as observed in patients, families, and caregivers (36). Such investigation would inevitably attend closely to the language used by sufferers to express their distress as revealing of the experience that underlies a particular form, rather than immediately translating the words into a biomedical idiom.

One of the nurses who participated in our nursing language study discussed previously provided us with a memorable example of the importance of attending to the actual language of a person who is suffering. This nurse told us of a woman, dying of cancer, who thrashed in bed apparently in agony, complaining of "burning." Treatments for first pain and then itching failed to provide any comfort. Only when the term "burning" was attended to within the context of the woman's religious beliefs was her distress recognized as spiritual in nature. The woman's vision of a hell that awaited her after death for an unresolved incident from her past ("a sin") was the cause of her suffering. A priest was sent for and the woman's agony was resolved.

Wilson's study of husbands' experiences of their wives' chemotherapy for cancer is an interesting example of an investigation that focused on the particular idiom of distress as a form of suffering, although not framed in the same terminology (34). In her grounded theory study, Wilson revealed and described the idiom of distress used by the husbands to talk about their "unrelenting nightmare." Understanding the three stages the husbands spoke about (identifying the threat, engaging in the fight, and becoming a veteran), advances clinical understanding of their suffering as well.

Building a literature of studies like Wilson's across forms of suffering is a strategy for creating an ongoing discourse on suffering for clinicians and researchers alike. Focus on the public manifestation or "routinized forms of suffering" will lead to understanding of the shared aspects of these human conditions (24).

As a fundamental human experience, suffering has a basic structure. To speak or write about a basic structure of suffering is to acknowledge a universal aspect of human nature. While each individual's suffering is unique, those aspects of being human that all people have in common lend a basic structure to the experience of suffering. This was evident in the BMT study by Steeves as compared to the nursing home study by Kahn (13), (14), (17). Knowledge of this structure would be useful for clinicians in assessing and working with suffering.

This assertion is perhaps less tentative and less surprising when the arguments phenomenologists have made about the lived world of human experience are considered. Phenomenologists have long pointed out that the human lived experience consists of four "existentials" or aspects that reveal the fundamental structure of the life world (37), (38). These essential aspects of humanness are the lived body or the experience of embodiment, temporality or the experience of time, lived human relations, and lived space.

We found in our research that suffering manifested in a way that included these four existential aspects in a three-fold dimensional structure. In other words, suffering disrupted each of these fundamental categories of human existence. More specifically, suffering altered our participants' experiences of embodiment, constricted, or radically changed and reduced, their social worlds in terms of human relationships and lived space, and changed their relationship with time. These dimensions can serve as a guide for the clinician's assessment efforts in that each dimension must be investigated in order to understand the totality of a person's suffering.

The experience of suffering involves the person in a larger process that includes the person's own coping with suffering and the caring of others. In the previous discussion of suffering and social interaction, we noted that suffering commences two related processes, one *intrapersonal* and one *interpersonal*. We illustrated this point with a basic triangular model. This model has developed with our work, and in its present form it appears as Figure 1–2.

In Figure 1–2, the basic structure of suffering as the apex of a triangle with caring and coping at the base remains, as does the assumption that suffering is a central experience that motivates and guides the responses of coping and caring. What has been added to this model are labels for the interactional processes themselves as we have come to understand them better through our work. For example, the relationship of suffering and coping describes the intrapersonal process of making meaning, which we described above.

Caregiving describes the interpersonal process of those efforts made by others to alleviate, ameliorate, or ease the person's suffering. In the case of nurses, for instance, such efforts include a repertoire that ranges widely from skilled interventions, to physical ministrations, to the use of technology, to therapeutic communication and so on. The point is that although nursing interventions are often aimed at specific symptoms or problems, they also impact and affect the larger issue of

FIGURE 1–2

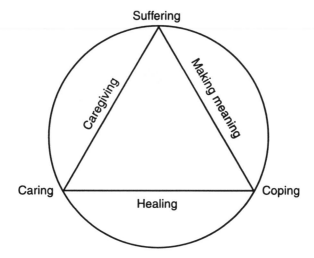

suffering. Caregiving occurs simultaneously with the intrapersonal struggle of the individual to make or find meaning. When both efforts are successful, the suffering of a person is balanced by healing.

The caring environment in which the processes of suffering occur can influence a person's suffering positively and negatively. While the responsibility of clinicians in caregiving is obvious, we must also attend more seriously to how the care environments influence the suffering of patients. It is important that clinicians begin to consider how care environments ameliorate suffering and also how they may interfere with the processes of making and finding meaning for each patient. Also, it is important to pay special attention to cases in which the organization of the delivery of care and cure services serves as a potential source of suffering for some patients and families. The case history of a "difficult" cancer patient detailed by Strauss and Glaser still stands today as one of the most poignant and horrible examples of this (39). These authors documented how the hospital staff's organized work environment led to the female patient's becoming increasingly isolated during her lingering and painful death in the hospital. These authors document how this isolation increased the suffering, or in their term "the anguish," she experienced in the hospital until her death.

Conclusion

The discussion above represents our best understanding of suffering to date based on our research, our clinical practice as hospice nurses, and the research and writing of others. Our understanding has grown through our work but much more needs to be done.

Nursing inquiry into suffering has just begun and there are a number of possible research directions. One possible direction—building a literature of description of forms of suffering—was mentioned above. The development of such a literature through case examples and qualitative inquiry would eventually allow for comparison and synthesis among forms of suffering. Our present work on suffering is proceeding in the direction of how culture shapes the experience and how cultural structures lend form to the meaning sufferers are able to make. We are focusing on groups that have strong traditions of suffering and enduring suffering, rooted in historical oppression, namely African-Americans, Appalachians, and Jews.

Also, more research is needed on how health care environments and health care delivery practices influence, interfere with, or enhance the experiences of patients within them who are suffering and attempting to make meaning of their suffering. Such research could focus on issues of health policy that promote increased risk of suffering.

Understanding suffering supplements the everyday practical knowledge needed by clinicians to care for individuals who suffer. An understanding of suffering provides a context of awareness for the professional caregiving that must take place in the clinical arena, placing our everyday work with these persons into a larger perspective. As suffering takes place at the level of the whole person, an awareness of it in our daily clinical practice centers us at the level of one searching human being reaching out to another. It is this level where our interventions must take place to be truly effective in a holistic way.

References

1. Kahn, D. L., & Steeves, R. H. (1986). The experience of suffering: Conceptual clarification and theoretical definition. *Journal of Advanced Nursing, 11,* 623–631.
2. Cassell, E. J. (1982). The nature of suffering and the goals of medicine. *New England Journal of Medicine, 306,* 639–645.

3. Spross, J. A. (1993). Pain, suffering, and spiritual well-being: Assessment and interventions. *Quality of Life, 2,* 71–79.

4. Benedict, S. (1989). The suffering associated with lung cancer. *Cancer Nursing, 12,* 34–40.

5. Bulger, R. J. (1992). Is our society insensitive to suffering? In P. L. Starck & J. P. McGovern (Eds.), *The hidden dimension of illness: Human suffering* (pp. 155–202). New York: National League for Nursing Press.

6. Loewy, E. H. (1991). The role of suffering and community in clinical ethics. *The Journal of Clinical Ethics, 2,* 83–89.

7. Rushton, C. H. (1992). Care-giver's suffering in critical care nursing. *Heart & Lung, 21,* 303–306.

8. Steeves, R. H., & Kahn, D. L. (1987). Experience of meaning in suffering. *Image, 19,* 114–116.

9. Kahn, D. L., & Steeves, R. H. (1988). Caring and practice: Construction of the nurse's world. *Scholarly Inquiry for Nursing Practice, 2,* 201–216.

10. Steeves, R. H., Kahn, D. L., & Benoliel, J. Q. (1990). Nurses' interpretation of the suffering of their patients. *Western Journal of Nursing Research, 12,* 715–731.

11. Kahn, D. L., Steeves, R. H., & Benoliel, J. Q. (1994). Nurses' views of the coping of patients. *Social Science & Medicine, 38,* 1423–1430.

12. Marris, P. (1974). *Loss and change.* London: Routledge & Kegan Paul.

13. Steeves, R. H. (1988). *The experiences of suffering and meaning in bone marrow transplant patients.* Unpublished doctoral dissertation, University of Washington, Seattle.

14. Kahn, D. L. (1990). *Living in a nursing home: Experiences of suffering and meaning in old age.* Unpublished doctoral dissertation, University of Washington, Seattle.

15. Gadow, S. (1980). Body and self: A dialectic. *Journal of Medicine and Philosophy, 5,* 172–185.

16. Sacks, O. (1984). *A leg to stand on.* New York: Harper & Row.

17. Steeves, R. H. (1992). Patients who have undergone bone marrow transplantation: Their quest for meaning. *Oncology Nursing Forum, 19,* 899–905.

18. Polkinghorne, D. E. (1988). *Narrative knowing and the human sciences.* Albany, NY: State University of New York Press.

19. Steeves, R. H., Kahn, D. L., Wise, C., Balwin, A. S., & Edlich, R. F. (1993). The tasks of bereavement for burn unit staffs. *Journal of Burn Care and Rehabilitation, 14,* 386–397.

20. Steeves, R. H., & Kahn, D. L. (In press). Family perspectives: The tasks of bereavement. *Quality of Life, 3*(3), 39–66.

21. Kahn, D. L., & Steeves, R. H. (In press). The significance of suffering for cancer care. *Seminars in Oncology Nursing, 11*(1), 1–75.

22. Cassell, E. J. (1991). *The Nature of Suffering.* New York: Oxford University Press.

23. Benoliel, J. Q. (1985). Loss and adaptation: Circumstances, contingencies, and consequences. *Death Studies, 9,* 217–233.

24. Kleinman, A., & Kleinman, J. (1991). Suffering and its professional transformation: Toward an ethnography of interpersonal experience. *Culture, Medicine, and Psychiatry, 15,* 275–302.

25. Shweder, R. A. (1988). Suffering in style. *Culture, Medicine, and Psychiatry, 12,* 479–497.

26. Arathuzik, D. (1990). Pain experience for metastatic breast cancer patients: Unraveling the mystery. *Cancer Nursing, 14,* 41–48.

27. Battenfield, B. L. (1984). Suffering: A conceptual description and content analysis of an operational schema. *Image, 16,* 36–44.
28. Brallier, L. W. (1992). The suffering of terminal illness. In P. L. Starck & J. P. McGovern (Eds.), *The hidden dimension of illness: Human suffering* (pp. 203–226). New York: National League for Nursing Press.
29. Charmaz, K. (1983). Loss of self: A fundamental form of suffering in the chronically ill. *Sociology of Health and Illness, 5,* 168–195.
30. Duffy, M. E. (1992). A theoretical and empirical review of the concept of suffering. In P. L. Starck & J. P. McGovern (Eds.), *The hidden dimension of illness: Human suffering* (pp. 291–303). New York: National League for Nursing Press.
31. Hinds, C. (1992). Suffering: A relatively unexplained phenomenon among family caregivers on non-institutionalized patients with cancer. *Journal of Advanced Nursing, 17,* 918–925.
32. Starck, P. L. (1992). The management of suffering in a nursing home: An ethnographic study. In P. L. Starck & J. P. McGovern (Eds.), *The hidden dimension of illness: Human suffering* (pp. 127–154). New York: National League for Nursing Press.
33. Twycross, R. G., & Lack, S. A. (1983). *Symptom control in far-advanced cancer.* New York: Pitman Books.
34. Wilson, S. (1991). The unrelenting nightmare: Husbands' experiences during their wives' chemotherapy. In J. M. Morse & J. L. Johnson (Eds.), *The illness experience: Dimensions of suffering* (pp. 237–314). Newbury Park, CA: Sage Publications.
35. Switzer, D. K. (1973). Human suffering in grief: Factors affecting intensity and morbidity. *Humanitas, 9,* 47–67.
36. Nichter, M. (1981). Idioms of distress: Alternatives in the expression of psychosocial distress: A case study from south India. *Culture, Medicine, and Psychiatry, 5,* 379–408.
37. Merleau-Ponty, M. (1962). *Phenomenology of perception.* London: Routledge & Kegan Paul.
38. Van Manen, M. (1990). *Researching lived experience: Human science for an action sensitive pedagogy.* London, Ontario: State University of New York Press.
39. Strauss, A. L., & Glaser, B. G. (1970). *Anguish.* Mill Valley, CA: The Sociology Press.

Chapter 2

Suffering in the First Person

Glimpses of Suffering Through Patients' and Family Narratives

"I'm More Than My Chart."

Nessa Coyle, RN, MS

Memorial Sloan Kettering Cancer Center

Author's Note

The following narratives were part of daily telephone conversations between a supportive care nurse and patients and families enrolled in the Supportive Care Program of the Pain Service at Memorial Sloan-Kettering Cancer Center in New York City. At the time these conversations took place, the words and phrases were recorded verbatim because of their resonance of depth of suffering. The words were spoken by old and young, men and women, married and single, rich and poor, educated and with limited education. All the patients had advanced cancer of various types. The common thread was that of suffering.

The narratives were selected randomly by the author, from a retrospective chart review, and cover a span of ten years. These selections do not purport to show a process or a resolution, they simply illustrate a depth of suffering that was expressed at that moment. The random selection brings out an emerging kaleidoscopic view which turns into an organized picture—a myriad of pieces that form a design of regular proportions and regular events.

Introduction

It is not only appropriate, but also important and even necessary to examine suffering from the words of those who suffer. The suffering of the dying and the suffering of their families is most often told in the words of others (1). Relating the actual words of patients and families spoken in the immediacy of the situation carries an urgency that words of others, charts, graphs, and diagrams cannot convey.

The privacy of suffering must always be expressed in the first person. Suffering is something that happens within a person—it is not observable. It may be deduced, inferred, and theorized but, in fact, only direct testimony communicates the suffering felt by an individual (2), (3).

When an individual gives life to his suffering by putting it into words he gives it a reality, a public existence that others may acknowledge and bear witness to. Communicating his private experience in this way, the sufferer may lessen his burden by sharing it.

We, the listeners, must realize that the words of the patients and families reveal the reality of their suffering, and hearing their words we carry this reality into public existence.

The narratives that follow are divided into three parts: those of the patients themselves, those of their families, and the narratives of bereavement after the death of the patient.

The themes of the patients' narratives—fear, loss, worry, despair, vulnerability, loneliness, the sense of being trapped, and of imminent death are powerfully revealed by the excerpts that follow. We are brought to an understanding on many levels—beyond tabulation, enumeration, and classification.

The families express the weariness and exhaustion of witnessing the decline of their loved ones, the loss of their lives as they knew them, and the terrible burden of responsibility that giving care places upon them.

When death interrupts their burden of responsibility and pain, the family members begin the process of forging a transition from one of the most difficult and challenging things they have ever done to some kind of normal life. The themes that emerge from the narratives of bereavement look backward to the death, the suffering, the relief experienced, the guilt experienced, all somehow coming together to give some meaning to their experience and to provide a means of transition back into life and the normal world of events.

The Patient: Despair, Loneliness, and Vulnerability

Despair, loneliness, and vulnerability are frequently encountered by patients with advanced cancer, as they struggle to come to terms with their disease. The rollercoaster of potential treatments or lack of treatments and dependence on and vulnerability to the health care system produces a weariness and anger in these patients, which often expresses itself in terms of despair, loneliness, and vulnerability.

Despair

The following excerpts show a sense of hopelessness and deep sadness.

> This whole place is a joke, no cure for this disease, I am 47 years old and have done nothing with my life, nothing.

> I may as well shoot myself.

> I woke up crying uncontrollable. I forgot I had cancer and then remembered.

I feel such sadness inside me I don't know what it is. I feel so sad, Nessa, something broke inside me.

I wonder if I should have surgery to get rid of the weight of the arm. Arms are like children, the brain the mother. Sometimes you have to sacrifice a child for the good of the whole.

Sometimes I don't care if I'm dead or alive. If things don't improve I'll put myself away. There's no way out.

(The following statements were made by a young man with a progressive brain cancer):

I sold my drums when I could no longer use the pedals. I loved those drums. Friends have let me down. If they call and I'm sleeping they don't call back. I hate that. I need my friends.

What's it all about? I'm seen as a tough guy but I'm not. I'm 31 and live with my mother but I need to be independent. I only know two speeds neutral and high gear. I'm having to adapt to a new way of dealing with things and it's hard. I can't walk. I can't go to the mall to buy presents. I sometimes have this feeling of rage around people.

I pray I won't wake up each morning. I want to feel good. I want to see the results from the chemo with my legs moving.

Nothing's going on. I'm just sick and tired of living that's all. (He shot himself that afternoon when his mother was out shopping.)

This sense of despair exemplified above seems often to stem from hopelessness about the diagnosis and the failure of repeated efforts to alter the disease or improve the quality of life.

Loneliness

The following words express the essential loneliness of suffering.

I've had a weekend of real fatigue and depression. It makes me feel very lonely, like there's no one who really understands what it's like, feeling that your options are running out. Cancer appearing all over the media, radio, TV, magazines, terminal cancer a major element, puts me into a gray, gray mood.

I miss my husband in bed next to me. I feel lost.

I feel so isolated. I'm an all or nothing person. I want to be able to walk like I use to, take care of my family like I use to, go out to eat like I used to. I can do nothing.

The above statements are reflective of the patient's sense of isolation and the feeling that one is alone in one's suffering and that no one can understand or share the pain.

Vulnerability

The suffering caused by having to rely on others in a previously self-sufficient individual causes great distress.

> If only doctors would listen to patients they would learn what is wrong.
>
> I have a sense of urgency about my care. That same urgency is not felt by the doctors and nurses.
>
> Surgery canceled for the second time. I wonder if my psyche will hold out.
>
> I'm too weak to come into the clinic, but I'd sure appreciate a phone call.
>
> My doctor is away. I expected to see him at the clinic. I feel betrayed.
>
> Each day the news louder and clearer. I'm reaching the point at which I am going to be totally paralyzed. Do you control the pain as the tumor is growing, do you become paralyzed, do I die from the tumor pressing against the spinal cord, what happens? Will I become bed-ridden for awhile in great pain, end up in an condition that they're having all those arguments about "right to die"? Has become a real issue for me. Euthanasia, right-to-die activists, keeps the subject before the public, I'm part of that public that's most keenly interested. It raises this TIME awareness, how overnight things can change.
>
> I feel this is a reprieve. I felt I was being kicked out of the nest at this stage of the disease.

These expressions are representative of the special vulnerability of patients with advanced cancer. They have been felled by their diagnosis, they have no means to do anything in their own behalf in actuality and little defense psychologically.

The Patient: Trapped

No way to win: Advanced cancer can leave patients in a trapped and vulnerable state knowing that they have no way to reach a desirable conclusion to their dilemma. They know they will die, and they know they will suffer, and they know that nothing can reverse this process.

Sometimes fear is the driving force for this feeling of being trapped. At other times, it is a treatment decision that results in no improvement with further pain and debility.

Treatment Disappointments

Treatment failures force a patient to confront the "realness" of the disease.

> I thought everything would be all right after surgery, I didn't expect this. I feel angry at what has been done to me.
>
> How can I now have extensive disease when I was told last month there were only a few cells left to wipe out?
>
> Sometimes I think about that second cordotomy, was it worth it, the trade off losing bowel and bladder function. But had to do it because of the pain.
>
> Was it worth it? I could walk before surgery. I have pain when I walk now. Was it worth all the pain and suffering, the operations and pain, was it worth it?

In each instance, the patient hoped for more than occurred. The cost–benefit balance was disappointing because it underscored and reinforced the sense that no matter what choice was made they were still trapped.

Trapped by Fear and Bewilderment

Finding oneself in a situation in which one sees no way out evokes fear.

> My roommate died. I heard her breathing and then no more. No one told me until I asked. I felt like running, running, running away but I couldn't.
>
> Lots of things going on right now. The tumor in my side is growing, something is going on in my back. I can only take things one at a time. I'm scheduled for a myelogram tomorrow. It was a bad experience last time so I'm scared. It's awful to be so frightened. I feel all beat up.
>
> What am I supposed to do? Lie back and die?

Talking about the fear and bewilderment lessened the anguish. Putting the fear into words gave it a form that could then be addressed.

The Patient: Loss

The losses suffered by patients with cancer come one on top of another with limited periods of respite over the course of their disease progression and treatment. The individual is often left depleted physically, psychologically, and spiritually. The following statements reflect frustration, anger, and resignation at these losses.

I have no control, my adulthood has been taken away from me. I'm told what to take and when, when I can and cannot go out. I make no decisions. No one knows how I feel. I want to learn what I can and cannot do through trying.

I feel cheated out of life. Life was supposed to begin at 40 and I got breast cancer. I feel deeply weary, heavy, exhausted. Any movement is so much effort.

I am not complete because my body does not function now. Before I was almost a normal person. Everything functioned even though I had pain for many years. I'm so impotent now I can't do what I want to. Yesterday my grandchild fell on a broom. I felt so bad I couldn't run to save her. I feel so inadequate in this world.

It scares me to see my arm so swollen. The girl (housekeeper) is scared at the size of my arm, so ugly. I suffer night and day. My life is ruined. That surgery three years ago, I feel it was forced on me. I feel I was abused. I feel so bitter. When I complained of pain I was made to feel a liar, like I am a pampered woman.

My life revolves around my bowels, whether or not I've had a bowel movement.

I am unable to do a thing for myself. I feel so frustrated. I need a person every second. I have nothing to wear. I will never be able to drive, like you cut off the wings of a bird. I am not strong enough to go places on my own. It is such a struggle to go out, so many clothes to put on so I turn down invitations.

For me frailty is a lot harder to bear than dying.

Things are tough. I'm starting to have difficulty in wiping myself. I'm scared about how this will effect my relationship with Joe. This decreased independence is driving me crazy.

Patients who are mourning the loss of life as it was, a body that one knew and could rely on, and adult status and control, suffer a diminished sense of worth. These losses are so overwhelming that the already exhausted patient is demolished even more.

The Patient: Worry

Patients worry about treatment decisions, the potential of being bed-ridden and a burden on the family, and financial resources being exhausted.

Decisions Regarding Treatment

Marked ambivalence and distress often accompany treatment decision making. More often, lack of ongoing treatment happens by default as the individual is too sick to tolerate it.

> I'm near the end psychologically, and then I have to make the decision whether to continue treatment or not. I live each day. I try and go along with the most up-to-date medical knowledge that will extend my life. I know my life is shortened. I think about death. I get frightened. I face death and ask the same questions as we all do ultimately. I try and live each day. I sometimes get panicky when I talk about it. I'm getting panicky now so we should stop.

> I'm frightened about going home. I don't do well with transitions. My legs are going rapidly, I can't support them. I have a heavy decision whether to have chemo or not. It's my decision because it's my body.

Decisions surrounding whether to continue treatment or not have a profound effect on the patient. On the one hand, continuation of treatment may result in some benefit, but with adverse side effects and increased debility. On the other hand, the decision to stop treatment implies acceptance of the futility of treatment and life's coming to an end.

Worry about Being a Burden

Worry about being a burden on the family is frequently reflected in patients' words.

> I wonder if my cancer is spreading. I wonder if I'm going to get better. I want people to be honest with me. I don't want to end up bedridden, incontinent, and a burden on my husband and family.
>
> I'm so fearful of the future, my disease spreading, being an invalid and a burden on my family. I remember the burden my mother was on me.
>
> I feel Annie is a burden on me and I am a burden on her. Maybe I should go into a retirement home. I would not like a nursing home.
>
> Sue would probably be better off if I wasn't around.
>
> John is under great stress. He's a doer, use to getting immediate results. Caring for me puts him in a very different situation from what he's use to.
>
> Who will take care of me so I don't burden my daughter? (after discussion about hospice care) I didn't think it was that bad.
>
> I see how fatigued Agnes is getting. I want her to go away for a weekend. I sometimes think of going into a veterans hospital.
>
> I don't want to destroy what I love. Sometimes I think of going into a place. When I first went home, the 18-month-old cried and demanded attention each time I needed help. Time was off, a year ago he wouldn't have fussed.

The thought of burdening one's family with the continuous grinding necessities of daily physical care is very upsetting to patients. They often foresee themselves in a bedridden, incontinent, highly dependent state. The worry about dragging down those one loves the most may make going to an in-patient facility a preferred option for some patients rather than being cared for at home.

Financial Worries

Concern about money generated high anxiety in patients as to whether their care will continue and be based on need or if it will be tailored to their resources.

> I'm worried about Medicaid renewal, if it doesn't go through my medications may not be covered. What would I do?
>
> I had a letter from my insurance. They are not paying the claims until further investigation. I am very worried.
>
> My husband is overwhelmed with all these bills. Before, I use to do them.

Why are they hounding me with the bills?

My insurance is being eaten up. There's no need for further tests.
If they find things there's not a hell of a lot they can do.

Financial concerns add to the stress of decision making and to
the general anxiety and uncertainty surrounding the disease and its
effect on their families.

The Patient: Fear

The days of many patients with advanced cancer are overshadowed by
fear. Fear of dying, fear of progressive debility, fear of a particular
symptom, and fear of abandonment. Not uncommonly, these fears are
magnified by night.

Acutely Feared Symptom or Disability

Patients fear a particular symptom or disability sometimes as much as
death itself.

A major fear is that I will experience the feeling of suffocation I
had before. I would rather die, be killed, than experience that again.

I'm afraid I'll be paralyzed. I'm afraid of a big infection. I'm afraid
they'll put tubes in me and keep me alive.

Meaning of life to me is my brain. Is the right of every individual
to commit suicide after consultation with a variety of people if in
desperate straits, that is no longer having a functioning brain. Not
at that state yet.

I'm afraid of falling when I'm alone. I'm afraid of going blind and
I'm afraid of being paralyzed.

I'm terrified. I can't move my legs. It terrifies me.

I'm terrified of choking to death. I have to talk about it.

I'm scared. Scared of the side effects of chemo, scared of losing my
hair, scared of dying and losing everything I loved doing. Before I
came right back after treatment but not now. I'm afraid that I am
no longer able to control the disease and the disease is beginning
to control me. I know all people go through this and I'm trying to
control it the best way I can.

Abandonment

Fear of abandonment by physicians, medical team, or loved ones can be expressed in softly spoken phrases tinged with great sadness and wistfulness.

> A long time ago I asked my boyfriend if he would take me in if things got really bad. He said "no, I will not be a caretaker."

> I'm so fatigued I'm afraid my boyfriend will abandon me. My arm is getting heavy. I can hardly use it, and what then? My voice is hard to project above a whisper. If I need less Percocet, it will show the Bismuth is effective.

> My boyfriend goes to functions on his own now that I can't go and that isn't good.

> At one hospital people didn't believe me. A terrible feeling when you know how you feel and can't convey that feeling to others. I feel my present doctors treat me like a man and appreciate what the disease has done to me.

> I wasn't invited anywhere for July 4th. I wouldn't have gone, but I would have liked to be invited.

> She didn't examine me very carefully, maybe she was tired or maybe she was indicating there was nothing more to do.

> I don't want to be transferred, I want to stay here to die, that's what I want. I don't want to have to go somewhere else. (Son pledged to father would make sure he stayed at Memorial, "his dying wish," and he did.)

> I can't understand what's happening to me, I'm not the same as I was before. I don't understand why my legs are swollen. I don't understand what's said to me, just words. I don't understand my medication. I'm not the same as I was before. You explain to me but I don't understand. You've been talking to my sister but I feel abandoned over the past few days.

These words echo a melancholy resignation that the patients see themselves as no longer existing in a meaningful way in the world.

Fear of Dying Yet Weary of Life

Fear of dying, yet weariness of life, may be the ambivalence expressed by depleted patients with cancer.

> I have such a fear of dying. I'm afraid that God is punishing me. I'm afraid of the pain. I'm afraid I will last longer because I feel

stronger. I want no tubes, no hospitalization. I'm afraid. Hospitalization is like a nightmare. I think I would lose my mind if I had to go through that again.

All these relatives visiting, it frightens me. They're coming just the way they did before my mother died. My time is easier than hers but I'm being given all these non-spoken messages that my death is near. It's difficult to live day by day.

I feel without hope. Sometimes I feel better, sometimes worse, but so weak. I don't know what is to be. Sometimes I feel each breath is going to be my last and I panic.

How do people die of cancer? How do people die of a heart attack? Wouldn't it be better for me? Shouldn't human beings be given the same option for euthanasia as animals?

Panic at the thought of death itself and how it will occur is not unusual. The unexpected visit by relatives who only visit at births, marriages, and funerals can be an abrupt confrontation with the reality of imminent death.

Fear of the Night

The quiet and darkness of night is a time when many patients feel the least protected. The distraction of daytime activity is absent, and the fears and anxieties that bedevil the patient come to the fore.

I'm afraid of sleeping. I'm afraid something imminent is going to happen. I want to know what's going on.

I had terrible anxiety during the night. Such anxiety I'll never be able to articulate to you. I really feel sympathy for the mentally ill.

I'm frightened at night. I don't know where I am. I'm not at home. I feel deserted and frightened. I dreamed I saw my daughter outside the window and I couldn't reach her. I'm afraid of never leaving the hospital. Of being entrenched here forever.

The days are so long. I'm afraid of going to sleep. If I shut my eyes when it is light I'm less scared.

I have these nightmares. Dead bodies. People and friends of mine who are dead.

Nights are hell. I get disoriented. I get so lost on the other (drugs) I just want to feel like myself again.

Nighttime fears often center around something catastrophic about to happen. Only by keeping awake can patients guard themselves from it.

The Patient: Wanting to Die

Expressions of wanting to die are seen here both as a response to immediate overwhelming pain and a response to progressive loss of function or feared further loss.

Pain: Immediate and Overwhelming

Immediate overwhelming pain obliterates all other sense data for the patient.

> The pain is terrible, help me, help me. Why don't you just kill me?

> The pain was so bad yesterday, if I had had a gun I would have shot myself. It's better now.

> Severe spasm of pain in the car. I felt like screaming, I stuffed Kleenex into my mouth to stop the sound coming out. I felt like opening the car door but I wouldn't do that to my husband.

> I want to be dead. Help me to die, that's all I want. I want to die. Why won't you help me?

> The patient screamed "Kill me, kill me" to her husband at the top of her voice, in the setting of sudden severe abdominal pain. After the pain was controlled, her words changed to, "I feel I am living."

The desperation caused by acute overwhelming pain is conveyed in these requests for death. When pain is relieved and suffering addressed, the requests diminish in frequency and intensity.

Loss of Hope: An Exhausted Spirit

The depletion of spirit by multiple losses makes death sometimes seem preferable.

> If people tell me that I am going to live for a very long time, I don't take it as good news. To die would be a liberation from my suffering.

I'm just waiting. I wish it would happen fast. Nothing is left for me, no living to do, nothing to put in order.

I want to die. I'm becoming demented. I can't write easily because of the weakness in my right arm. I feel Beth wants me to stay alive as a vegetable.

I know I'm at the end of the road so what's the point. My wife may as well put me away in a nursing home. When I knew there was a tumor down there I knew it was the end. I've worked all my life, worked since I was 12, I knew the Depression, I was going to retire this year. I ask God to take me away and not make me suffer.

I'm having to learn how to live with this thing, it's not going away.

I don't want to become a vegetable with tubes and things.

Whenever all of you are tired, it's OK to bow gracefully out, I'm ready. I don't want to be resuscitated. I thought of not coming into the hospital last night but too hard on Beth.

How long does this dying take, I want to pack it in. I'm sleeping, not living, I'm constipated.

Every night I go to bed hoping that I won't wake up in the morning. I have no will for life, this is not my country.

I want to die I can't live like this, I can't move my left arm and I'm afraid of losing my right arm. I can't stand the reality of not being able to move my arm.

If I say I want to live I'm lying. I should feel grateful to God, Russ and the children are healthy. I ask God to have compassion on me, my spirit is poor. The impotence. I saw bulbs in the greenhouse and tried to replant them, I made such a mess, it made me feel so bad, so impotent.

You are one person talking to a friend, listening to their animated conversation, then pain strikes, and like a switch you are someone else, with the pain in a flash it isn't me any more.

I'm afraid that the sharp spasms of pain will become prolonged, death must be better than that.

My greatest fear is of increased pain. Greater than of death.

I've wanted to kill myself at times but haven't had the courage. It's not just the pain, it's the whole situation. I had hoped I would die on the table. That would take care of everything, no struggle.

My life's work is done but I'm not able to die, how can the day-to-day time I have left be given a sense of meaning. The hardest thing is living without a goal, a new way of being, just being, that's the hardest thing.

It's not the dying that's hard, but living in a weakened state.

How will I die? What will it be like? I fear the unknown. I feel such enormous sadness. There are so many things undone. How will the disease progress? My legs are numb. They always told me to watch out for that.

I've thought of suicide and yet I love life. It's boring and a chore to be sick. I'm afraid of starving to death. I'm afraid of losing Lucy. I'm deeply in love with life and I'm deeply in love with my wife and I want to retain that state of being. Lucy gave me hope. I'm afraid I won't like the food she makes and she will be disgusted. Life depends on eating. I'm afraid people are planning my death and not telling me about it. I'm scared shitless. I'm an anxious person. I've felt the void and emptiness of not existing. Fear is based on the abstractness of life. I haven't dealt with my son's death yet.

I know I'm going to die at some point, but I don't want it to be an undignified and painful death. This is the most important time in my life and yet I feel disconnected from it. I feel disconnected from the universe. I use to meditate, look at the moon and meditate, but now I am so focused on trying to position my arm and moving so I don't get a bedsore I'm unable to think of deeper issues.

Ambivalence about death sometimes lessens as patients become more and more frail. The hope becomes one for a dignified and merciful death.

Patients: Summary

The patients' words reflect fear, despair, and vulnerability, the rollercoaster of emotions as hopes of treatment success rise and are dashed. In their vulnerable state, the patients worry that they will be abandoned by an overwhelmed family or uncaring health care system. The power of the suffering and distress in these statements is revealed in the patients' expressions of feeling trapped. Requests for early death and requests for placement in a nursing home are statements of ultimate despair.

The Family: Burden of Care

Most of the burden of care of patients with advanced cancer is carried out by families in the home. Dealing with the patient's symptoms, giving medications, helping with daily activities, such as bathing and eating, all fall on the shoulders of the family members.

Home Care—Responsibilities and Exhaustion

Families become exhausted by attempting to meet both the needs of the patient and the needs of the family as a whole. These statements reflect the resultant irritability and stress.

> Everything's such a production. Everything takes so long. To eat, to dress, everything.

> I'm afraid to leave her alone. She might fall or have an angina attack. I feel guilty if I go out for any length of time. She tells me to go and then asks me why I've been so long. I've taken over the woman's work in the home, cooking and cleaning. She has too much pain and is too sick to do it.

> Others look forward to the weekend, but I dread them.

> I get angry with Barry. He doesn't take responsibility for things. I have to remind him to take his pills, to drink. He has to be coaxed to eat. I want to talk to him about dying, about funeral arrangements, what he wanted and everything. He just closes his eyes as though I'm not there.

> I'm doing all right, I get frustrated. I feel I have to make all the decisions and I guess that's the way it should be. But I take care of one thing and something else occurs. I can't achieve what I want to. I have all the means but I still can't do it. I hope I'm doing all that I can for Norma because that's what I have to live with.

> I'm so torn. My husband is sick, my baby is little, who do I take care of first? Both are calling me, who do I go to first?

> I feel exhausted. Constant demands on me from my boss, husband, and demented half-sister. George expects me to do everything. He doesn't want others to do it. If I go out, he waits for me to come back before catheterizing himself. When I come through the door he asks for things even though the house is full of people. I'm beginning to resent it. If he loves me he should think of me.

> This is all such a burden on me. I can't sleep, can't eat. I feel I'm cracking up. I can't cope. I'm the one who is here all the time. Had to do the income tax, have to dash out to shop and dash home. His brothers stay for a while and then say good-bye, good luck. My niece has her own life to lead. Everyone is getting tired. They have their own lives to lead.

> They didn't hear me. This isn't going to work if I can't bring him into the hospital if I have to.

I can't stand it any more. I'm trapped, overwhelmed. My older daughter is acting up. I'm waiting for something catastrophic to happen. I'm not able to leave the house. I'm trapped by his fear of my going out and my fear of going.

I'm like a dishrag. I go into the house, shake, cry, look at her. I'm afraid when I go down the avenue she won't be still alive. Nothing is normal anymore. You don't act normal around her. Even the kids act more formal. Everyone is panicked. Everyone's sitting around waiting for the next pain, the next symptom. I hear the phone ring and I say "Oh my God what's happened?" Nothing's the same, everything's a downer. A neighbor called and said she was praying for her to die.

Is it hard for him? Does he have pain? When I spoke to him he said, "help me" then nothing more. His eyes are open and yet he doesn't see.

Janie follows me around all the time. I think she is asleep and I leave to do something and she's right behind me. I would like her to be at peace with herself that's all.

Unless the health care system provides adequate support for the families of symptomatic patients being cared for at home, misery is the result for both the family and the patient. The words of the families send a powerful message.

Home Care—Watching Deterioration

The emotional turmoil of watching a family member change from a vibrant interactive person to a debilitated dependent individual takes its toll, as reflected by these statements.

Each day sucks for me, hard to get up. I'm just watching him waste away, only his spirit left. It's so hard. I just don't like to see it happen. Hard to watch. Even though we have wonderful friends I'm the one who sits and watches him each day.

My mother is so demanding and difficult, wants us to be there all the time. It's been going on for so long, it shouldn't happen to a dog. I've come to realize this is not my mother anymore. The prolonged illness and pain has changed her over time. She's jealous of the mobile. That was never my mother.

If it was me, I think I would have killed myself. I feel strongly about that. They even allow animals to be put out of their misery.

I've been floating on that long dark ocean all on my own for the past month. He's not in pain, just fading away. The doctor says make him more comfortable. I don't know what that means. Does it mean give him an enema, milk of magnesia, Tylenol?

It's hard, not getting any better. He's pretty much confined to his bedroom, the bed or chair, oxygen-dependent. He listens to music and reads. Sometimes there's gutteral sounds coming from his room. I'm afraid he's in pain but he said not. He's taken the phone out of his room and has stopped seeing friends. That's the way he wants it.

I wish she was the way she used to be, walking with a cane, out two to three times a week. It's a pathetic case. We are all exhausted. I've lost ten pounds. I go to the hospital each day to feed her. Her daughters are exhausted. We all travel to the hospital each day.

I get so worried with the long weekend coming up and people being away. His legs are like sticks. I had my nephew, the doctor, come and see him.

The following quotation is the most poignant summary of this anguish.

There is such emotional turmoil in caring for a sick person at home. The decision-making, a reactive approach, not sure if doing right or wrong, not wanting to harass people. Bert is a different person. He used to be highly animated, bright and energetic, giving to others in an unusual way, loving to talk. Now he seems a shadow of himself, sometimes not Bert at all.

Home Care: Own Needs Not Being Met

Totally sacrificing one's own needs to the needs of others can cause anger and resentment when prolonged.

It's so hard. I'm not a nurturer. That's why I didn't have children. I have no time to do anything for myself. Tom gets angry with me. I'm separated from my art. I always said that would kill me. I'm dying piece by piece.

My father does not really know what's wrong with him. He should really know but it's my mother's decision not to tell him. My mother's having such a hard time. She's used to being out and around. It's a burden on her, depressing and hard, but guilt would not let her place him in a nursing home.

Jim's world view is narrowed to focus on his immediate needs and TV. My needs and the children's are much wider. I deeply care for Jim, but the strain is great.

I have a feeling of suspended animation, waiting for something to happen. It's difficult to continue to live actively and engage with each day. I'm overwhelmed with sadness. It's all so sad. My birthday was on May 31st. He didn't remember. There are no celebrations. The holidays are coming up. Last year we went away. A couple years ago our dog dropped dead on my birthday. It could happen to people that way too.

These people suffer a double loss. They are giving more than ever before and have ceased to receive whatever support and joy they had been accustomed to before. Now their needs always take second place.

"I Don't Want to Take Him Home"

Fear of responsibility in caring for a dying family member, feeling pressured to do so, and not knowing what to expect may provoke violent anger from families.

(When discharge planning was discussed with the wife of a very debilitated man, her immediate response was): "If I have to take him home I'll kill him and kill myself." She then started to participate in planning for him to go home.

Talking about hospital beds, and Hoyer Lifts, don't they understand I can't care for him at home. It would kill me. I want him in a hospital.

"I'm worried about Angelica. She's still asking that I take her home, but it's too hard. I have my own medical appointments. I can't take care of her all the time."

It's important for families to be able to express their anguish at the prospect of taking someone home. Getting it out in the open gives them the ability to sort out whether or not they can, or will, be care givers.

The Family: Uncertainty

Uncertainty, frequently the hallmark of cancer in general and of treatment outcome, is difficult for families to deal with.

Uncertainty About the Goals of Care

The suffering and stress of families is increased by uncertainty and mixed messages from the medical team regarding the goals of care.

I'm not sure where he's going. Is he living or dying?

I'm frightened. I feel as though I'm on a time bomb.

I'm so confused. On one hand I am told Ben will probably be dead in 6–8 weeks. On the other hand further chemo is being planned in 3 weeks. I'm scared about him going home. What would I do in emergency situations? what would they be? how will he die? If it is heart failure, how will that be?

John is spending most of his time in bed. He thinks he is dying and I'm bewildered by it. I've been told that his X-rays and blood work are good.

He seems to have this terrible anger. I wonder if he is having a nervous breakdown. He refuses to walk much, to do exercises, to eat. He tries to sleep during the day and is up and down all night.

I don't know what to expect. Will the pain get worse and worse? Will he have to take more and more pills? It's so pathetic to see him.

The medical treatment offered implies an expected outcome. Families are often confused about whether to expect a death soon or some prolongation of life.

Home or Hospital as the Place of Care?

The family's decision on where someone will die is often surrounded with great anxiety.

I may be able to manage. But I panic. I get into a state. My mother died a year ago of cancer in Florida. It was awful.

I want him to be at home when he dies but what am I going to do? I want him to die at home but I don't know what to do when he talks about his funeral clothes, what he wants to wear, about cremation.

My major worry in taking him home is uncertainty of nursing coverage.

Should I quit work and stay home? I don't like to stay at home, that bothers me, but I feel I should be with him if he hasn't much time left.

I don't know what to do. I've never cared for someone who has been ill. I don't know whether he should have radiation therapy near home or come back to Memorial where he knows the system. He has never been sick before, has never had pain before.

I can nurse him to life. I cannot nurse him to death. He is lost to me now.

Past experience with death, desire to care for someone at home, security with medical and nursing support all make the decision to care for someone at home easier.

The Family: Loss

Loss of life as it was, the person I knew, a future together and most sadly, hope, are shown in the following family statements.

Loss of Life as It Was

Diminution of the patient's life to one of dependence and limited interaction causes sorrow to the family.

I have trouble dealing with his passivity, his growing dependency on the nurse, the life of an invalid.

Life is almost down to TV dinners.

I can't believe all of this. Eight months ago she was well, we were having a good time. Now she is lying there, her eyes open, hallucinating. She didn't sleep last night. She lay there talking to herself. She didn't seem to be in pain.

I'm overwhelmed with the rapidity of it all; two weeks ago he was shoveling snow.

This loss of life as it was may be gradual or sudden, but even for those people whose losses have been gradual and cumulative the realization of the loss may be abrupt.

Loss of Hope

The realization both that there is no hope and that the loved one is not going to recover creates questions about the ability to continue to care for the person, as well as generating deep sadness.

It's much more difficult planning her death than planning, working to keep her alive.

It's very difficult for me to see her this way. It's very difficult for me to go into her room. It brings my mother's death back to me. I was ten, my brother was six, it was terrible. I was brought up by my father. It was very difficult for me. This brings it all back.

I see the reality of a very sick man rather than one being discharged to convalesce.

There is a deep sadness on both our parts. He will probably get no better than he is at present.

I'm beginning to face up to the reality of my sister's dying. I was blind before. How could I have missed it? I should have spent more time with her. I'm afraid of her dying. I'm afraid to bring it up to her. Death is a hard thing to talk about. Maybe I should take a leave of absence or take a part-time job.

It's killing me watching her but I'm glad she's at home. We haven't talked yet about dying but we both know.

I've given up hope. I cry no more. Once I learned he had a brain tumor nothing was left. It's awful to live without hope. I wish it was over all ready for both him and for me. He has lost his spirit. It's no fun for him watching family members catering to him, being screwed because of him.

When families lose hope, they start to accept their loss and begin the process of bereavement.

Loss of the Person I Knew

There is often a need to convey to others who this person was before having been ravaged by illness. In some ways, that also defines who the family member is.

She's losing her memory. She's very bright you know, has a PhD in music. I think she wants to stay at home at the end.

My wife is a different person than before. Like an empty drum. I go out sometimes and feel guilty. I'm torn between priorities—her and my work.

I felt an intense sadness as I looked at her. Something vital in her has been eroded by drugs, by pain, by the disease.

It's hardest for me when he doesn't respond, isn't lucid. When he talks to me and is lucid I zero in on that person.

I see him as a wounded animal. I cannot think of him in terms of the man I married and lived with for so many years and with whom I shared so much. It would rip me apart. I know tears are cathartic but I have to function. We went to Europe, he in a wheel chair. Frustrating not being able to see all the things I wanted to see. It was a horror seeing his humiliation with his weakness, having to crawl on his hands and knees in a cab to get to the door.

He doesn't read. His quality of life is dropping off to sleep over TV. I don't know if buying time was worth it. Time, sleeping, quality of life. I watch him die inch by inch, getting thinner and thinner, not able to turn. If it was me I would have wanted to take my own life but wouldn't have out of fear of being damned.

My husband is at a deeper level of depression than before. He has no inner resources. He tends to be a denier but he can't deny when he sees life vanishing, disappearing before his eyes, his professional life and actual life. He talks of dying, that he's dying although the doctor says he is not actively dying.

A history together of sharing thoughts, activities and memories, which make up a sense of one's identity, may be lost as debility increases.

The Family: Death

The conflicts and ambivalence about death are reflected in the words of these family members who express, on the one hand, fear of the dying process, and on the other hand the desire for death to come quickly. More conflict is engendered when patients request euthanasia or assisted suicide.

Fear of the Dying Process

The experience of caring for a dying relative at home makes one confront death.

I'm afraid of him dying. It's not an everyday occurrence you know.

I don't know what to do. I'm frightened. I'm here all alone. My son stayed until 11 PM. We were afraid something might happen, like him dying. I've never seen anyone actually die. My mother died at home. I remember her lying in the bed, sickly, I was about 14 years old. My father died in the hospital. We were just going to see him and he passed away. We just missed him. Mr. G. told me last night, "The walls are closing in on me." He's getting rough with me. He doesn't want to take his pills. I tell him he must or he will get terrible pain.

I'm keeping away from there, death isn't easy. The children are coming home this weekend. I told my daughter to bring a dark dress. It will all be over soon. I'm ready for her to die.

Nothing good is happening here. He is about to die, the clock is ticking. I don't know what to expect, how long it will last.

What's the use of her rallying so she will just have to suffer again?

Her body is swollen. She talked about dying last evening. What's the point of her life being prolonged for 2–3 months just to suffer? I'd like it over and done with. Her arms are so thin. It's OK when I don't talk about it but when I do I get all choked up. The funeral arrangements are made, it'll cost about $6,000, but what can you do?

Participation in death as a caregiver can be very frightening because one wants to do everything right and not make mistakes. This fear can be so extreme that family members must absent themselves from the room of the dying patient.

Wanting Death to Come Soon

Wanting death to come soon is often experienced in the setting of a lengthy, debilitating illness and prolonged dying process. It generates feelings of guilt.

I feel guilty for saying it but I wish it was over. I think that she's worried about us.

His friends wish him dead because it's too painful to see him in that state, and they wouldn't want to be in that state. Jim himself has not asked to be killed. But when I asked him what do you want to do today, he said "to die." I asked him if he wanted me to stop feeding him (tube feeds) he said no.

He's not making an effort. I don't want to push him anymore. He's had a long fight and it is time to rest. It's not a failure, it's a choice, a rational choice.

I wish it would happen fast and get it over with. I feel guilty for saying it but I wish it was over.

He's suffered too long. Maybe he'd be better off dead. Maybe he's been dead for the past 15 months. Taking all those pills and only about an hour's pain relief.

We're all psyched up for her to die. Psyched up that she's not going to make it. If she does it'll be a miracle. I don't want her to go on living will all this pain. If she goes under I don't want her to be resuscitated. Her spirits are nil. She's in and out of a trance.

> She had a neuro exam yesterday, questions about time and place. She was very upset by that. Today she kept preparing herself for the next exam. Kept repeating "March is after February, isn't that right, Joe?"

Bearing witness to the suffering of a dying loved one, and the exhaustion of continuous care giving contribute to a sense of futility, pointlessness, and wanting it to end. Guilt and ambivalence are swept away by the exhaustion.

Conflicts over Requests for Assisted Suicide

When a loved one is asked by a dying friend or relative to hasten death, it creates a dilemma.

> Tom has spoken to his lawyer about it. It would be an ethical dilemma if he ever asked me to do it. He talks of suicide but not often. But is he able to clearly make that choice? He's so drugged out. What if he suddenly wakes up and realizes his predicament? We agreed a long time ago that each would help the other end it all. He would not want to live like this. How long will it go on?

> Jennie wants to pack it in. She wants me to help her, but is worried how she could do it without harming me. Her biggest fear is time. She's giving away her clothes and jewelry.

The requests of a dying person are usually considered a sort of moral and social duty to fulfill. The one request that gives pause, and rests on the conscience of the caregiver, is that for assisted death. The request for assisted suicide from a dying patient is perhaps the one request that most threatens the family.

The Family: Summary

These statements from families illustrate their turmoil in caring at home for a symptomatic patient with advanced cancer while trying to work and run a household. Conflict and distress are everywhere: they become afraid to go out in case something happens, but can't bear staying in. They dread the weekends when few people may be around and worry about their decisions surrounding care. They are torn between whose needs are greatest within their family. Exhaustion may lead to making demands on the patient that are greater than can be realized. The family member can't sleep and keeps an ear open at night in case the sick person needs something. The distress increases if the patient seems distressed and uncomfortable with poorly controlled symptoms, which the family are forced to witness, cannot escape from, and feel responsible for, in that what they are doing is not bringing relief. If an escape is not available (such as a hospital admission if it is wanted), the family becomes overwhelmed.

Bereavement

The following statements made by husbands, wives, brothers, sisters, sons, and daughters were selected randomly at different stages of bereavement. The family members' words exemplify eight different themes: the struggle to reconstruct a life; coming to terms with the void left by the death; relief at the death; search for meaning and purpose in the dead one's suffering; mythifying the dead one; coming to terms with the guilt of things done or not done; recounting the dying process; and reliving the loved one's suffering. These themes all form an effort to make a transition to resuming life.

Finding a Transition

The families' struggles to come to terms with their experiences in caring for a loved one who died and to go forward with their lives is shown in the following narratives.

> I'm trying to be young again. To feel young again.
>
> I'm working very hard. Very involved trying to complete Gillian's work. A way of trying to keep her near to me, but it's not really working. We had so much in common, it was the first time both really in love.
>
> I'm sort of lost. I'm doing the laundry. Jamie is angry but I expect there will be a lot of that.
>
> I feel numb, in and out of the twilight zone. I don't know what it is to be a widow. I don't want to know. I don't know what a distraught wife is, my husband didn't want me to be sad. I refuse to act bereaved and sit on a sofa.

Sometimes I don't have any feelings about Judy. That makes me feel, if you're dead that's it. My father died and life went on and I felt—is that all there is?

I'm becoming overwhelmed, the upkeep of the house, the boiler broke, mowing the lawn. I'm having to make choices for the first time in my life. It's so hard, where to live, where to go, what to do. I'll need an accountant, a tax man, a lawyer.

I spend 60–65 percent of my time thinking of Sue, reminiscing. I like to spend time with people who knew both Sue and me. I'm closest at present to those who were part of her illness and dying.

I can't believe the reality of her death. I'm trying to find structure to my life. The babies are both a support and a wonder.

It's very hard. People keep coming into the store not knowing Peter's dead. I have not yet had to deal with living alone. That's to come.

I'm beginning to realize she really went. I feel comfortable in the house. I feel she's around or will come back. I miss her most when I go out. Then I feel very alone, especially at the weekends. My daughter comes to see me once or twice a week and brings me food for the week.

I've bonded with Saul's soul brother, I felt the transference when we shook hands at the wake. Saul was half-dead when he received the last rights, his eyes flickered half open as he said the Our Father with the priest, conversed only once more after that for ten minutes. It was unbelievably beautiful. His diaries show his struggle for life and independence in the knowledge of pending death.

Still absorbed by the experience of caring for a dying relative, the families have their emotions in two places—with the deceased and with their responsibilities to life.

The Void

The sense of emptiness left by the death of someone who was an integral part of one's life is expressed by families as a tangible void.

It's so hard. There's a great big hole in my heart. I miss her terrible. I'm seeing a psychiatrist.

I am so lonely, I miss him so. When I passed through the room he would say "Do you have a hug for me" and I always did. Michael talked over a long period of time of wanting to die. I can't be sorry that he's dead, but he suffered so much. Life is so empty without him, he was my favorite child. I gave Michael so much of my life and he gave so much to me. He knew all about guns, he took a course in his teens, his father was a hunter, but Terry didn't like killing anything. Michael made the guns secure last year when we were afraid his father might kill himself. Michael looked so peaceful, all the pain lines were gone from his face. I felt good about that. I don't know what I'll do yet when the family leaves.

Look what happened to me, Nessa. She was a most wonderful woman. Look what happened to me.

Stunned is the right word. Surprised I feel this way. I knew all along that Tim was terminal, but it's different when it happens. All my day was planned around Tim. Suddenly the void. I cried very hard for one and a half days, now I don't know how I feel.

I feel as though part of me has been ripped out, I thought the sun might cure her. How primitive we are, how near to animal we are.

I'm having a hard time, much harder than I thought I would. I can't get Joan out of my mind. I can't sleep at night. I had so much to do when Joan was sick, I was so involved. Now there's an emptiness. The nights are the hardest.

I'll miss him every hour of my life.

The nights are still hard. I hear him calling me, jump up, and find he's not there.

People say there's a void or emptiness when someone dies. That's not true, there's an intense presence all the time. I'm living with a dead man.

There is such a void in my life, and a part of me is gone and forever will be with my John. Everyday of the past year was devoted to my John and I just can't believe he doesn't need me anymore.

It's very tough on Bill (her father had been married 58 years) he just sits around, thinks about her, and cries. She was a giant and we miss her.

Families experience a violent wrenching loneliness, and think constantly about the deceased—thinking the person is still there and then facing the realization that he or she is gone.

Relief That It's Over

The extent of the family member's exhaustion by daily care and bearing witness to prolonged suffering is reflected in these expressions of relief at the ordeal's end.

A sense of relief that it's all over. I realized in the end only a miracle would give Martha back her health. Martha was not afraid of dying but not able to understand the suffering. But all the saints suffered. It's not understood until later.

Numb but all right. I'm glad he's not suffering anymore. I cry because he was dying. I cry because he's dead.

I don't wake up anymore looking for him. I got rid of all of his clothes and cried over each one of them.

(Mrs. P. burst into tears) He died at 8:15 PM. It's an incredible relief. Sense of relief but also of great sadness. He so much didn't want to die.

The suffering, superimposed on exhaustion that was experienced by both the patient and family, is resolved by death—a bittersweet resolution, tinged with guilt for the surviving family.

Mythifying the Dead One

Speaking of the dead one not in terms of suffering, but in terms of existence after death, of courage, and of being with them still are seen in these words.

I almost picked up the phone to call you yesterday. I had a dream with Marta in it. She said hello to you. She looked happy and well. I use to be very afraid of death but now I have no fear, not the same person after an experience like that. I'm not afraid of death. When it comes it comes. I might even welcome it. I keep her ashes with me. Where I go, she goes too.

I didn't think she wanted to die with me looking at her. I turned my back and she died. You brace yourself for it to happen, but it's still a shock.

While everything was going on, the dog ate his supper, went into his kennel, put down his head, and died. We'd had the dog for 14 years.

It all happened so fast, the death and funeral. So much to do little time to think. I saw my mother the Saturday before she died, my mother did not seem to recognize me. She kept on asking me what the time was, "because Jesus is waiting for me." I wasn't prepared even though I knew. I had never experienced a close death before.

Difficult over Thanksgiving and Jennie's birthday. She was born in November and died in November. Holiday season is difficult. Jennie bought presents for us all, last gifts. I still wake up at 8 AM and 5 PM, time for Jennie's medication. Also I sometimes think I have to do this or that, and then realize I don't have to anymore.

I sometimes feel Jennie's presence, had sort of hoped that would happen. Not scary.

I talk to George all the time. Before he died he told me never to feel alone, we'd always be together, I could always talk to him. He always used to say to me, take care of Tim first and then of me. He wanted Tim to have a car for Christmas. I want to get him that.

This was the first time I have ever kissed a dead person. I wasn't afraid, I loved him. I know no harm would come to me from him. I couldn't go back into the room until they had taken the bed away. I still can't believe that year. I was actually glad when he died, not in pain. He went out quietly. I and the nurse were with him, our sons were upstairs.

I feel grateful and elated that over the past two years we did everything we could. My courage helped her and her courage helped me. I slept in the same bed with her to the end. I was her advocate as she would have been mine. Overall it was a good death although her pain and anxiety increased towards the end. I did everything possible. I rose to the occasion. She's inside me to a great extent. I keep her urn in the bedroom. I talk to her as normal. Not morbid or clinging to the past but integrating past and present.

These narratives reflect a sense of continuity and reflection rather than turmoil, anxiety, and exhaustion.

Search for Meaning and Purpose

Questioning the reason for such suffering before death is seen in these narratives.

We're all taking it hard. It didn't dawn on me she was that sick. She never complained. So many questions left unanswered, why it happened and how, she was so careful.

I shouldn't have signed for surgery. It's driving me crazy. I watched him, took care of him, and in just one hour he was gone. He died and I am dying slowly. I did everything day and night, I had a purpose, I was hoping. I have no purpose. I keep thinking why, why, why. That "why" is going to kill me. The days he ate better I said "what does the medical profession know, he'll be all right." Maybe I lived in a fantasy world, but when you've lived together for 51 years you hope. Not only did he die but I think I'm dying. I can't find no consolation. After taking such care of him to come to this. He died and I am dying. I don't know if I have the right to blame myself. He would have died a natural death, he was getting sicker. I was occupied, I had what to do. Now I open the door and I am alone.

Sometimes I wake up with crazy thoughts. Why did she have to suffer like that? Sometimes thoughts tempt me. The crazy pain she went through, for what? Why did she have to suffer like that? You sort of warned me it would be hard. I guess it's true. I thought before you were talking about someone else. Now I realize you were talking about me.

His breathing seemed so hard, it must have been hard for him. Dr. S. is a Christian man. He says if there's a straight line to God, Chris gets it. He suffered more than Jesus Christ.

By finding an explanation for the loved one's suffering and death, the family gives a form and shape to the event, which fits into their view of the world.

Guilt for Things Done or Left Undone

The words of these families show how responsible they feel for decisions made prior to the loved one's death.

It would have helped if I'd understood the cause of his agitation and delirium. I regretted the feeding tube put in the last admission. Dr. S. said he didn't want him to starve to death. We didn't use it in the last two weeks. My family are still with me. I haven't yet started my new life.

If I had got him help earlier it would not have gone on for so long. Depression is no stranger in our house.

I had an initial high, everything was done with such love. But now at a low ebb, maybe I wasn't sensitive enough, maybe I could have done more. Two years ago I didn't want to be around sickness, I wanted to have fun. I was thinking more about me.

I can never forgive him for saying that, for saying "help me Jess to get out of your way." How could he say that, as though I wanted to get rid of him.

Berkley was interested in me for a long time. I wouldn't go until they found a spot for Jessica. They did two weeks ago. I only regret I didn't know how bad her liver chemistries were a few weeks ago. I could have spoken to her about which projects were most important for her to complete.

My only regret was that mother was so ashamed of her disfigurement by the disease.

She went downhill so rapidly after they took her off the experimental drug. I'm not sure if there was a connection. I'll send you her records of when she was at home. It may help others.

Worry that different decisions might have led to a different outcome are hard for the family to deal with.

Recounting the Dying Process

These unadorned words show vividly the starkness of witnessing a difficult death.

At the end the pain was terrible, not controlled. Morphine injections didn't help. Then she just folded her hands, laid back her head, and died. On Sunday we had a good time. Her life was music.

Four days before he died he had seizures, three days of hell, didn't rest for three days and nights. I feel badly about the end, it wasn't handled well. (He died in hospital.)

People were very supportive when I came to the hospital. It was difficult seeing him with an oxygen mask on his face. I was angry about seeing the respirator in the room. It was horrible for me, for my in-laws, for my children. I don't know how horrible it was for Mathew. My anger is beginning to abate but its still there.

I'll miss her a lot. I lived with her for the past two years. I was with her when she died. The last half hour was very hard. She kept reaching over and touching my face. Her breathing was a problem. She kept pulling her oxygen mask off saying, "I can't breathe, I can't breathe." She died 5–10 minutes after a shot. I wonder if she would have died if she hadn't had the shot. Her head tilted to one side. She was looking at me with eyes open not breathing, took a couple of breaths, reached out to touch my face as though to say "Don't worry, stay with me, touch me." Felt pressured by the autopsy request. It was very upsetting when I said she's been through enough, suffered enough, and the doctor saying, "She won't feel anything." I felt we were speaking a different language, communicating on different levels.

It's harder instead of better at the moment. The hardest part of my mother's last 24 hours was hearing her difficulty breathing, waiting for the last breath to come, wanting the last breath to come. Also struggling with her sometimes when changing her "Depends" as though fighting her. Also sometimes her hands reaching out as though she wanted something.

I couldn't believe it. I was on the telephone and saw his chest wasn't moving. He told me this morning he loved me. I loved him so much. He told me he couldn't hold onto the rope any longer.

I told him, "I know." I told him just to sleep. The children were in the garden playing.

The most difficult period was when he was actively dying. He abruptly awakened, seemed to panic, kept pressing the rescue button and said give me more, give me more. After the Ativan he went into a deep sleep and didn't awaken again.

Slept in mother's room the night she died. Would have been frightened if the nurse had not been there. I thought she had died several times. Long period without breathing and then she would take another breath.

She talked in whispers for the last 48 hours, never shut her eyes. Agonizing to watch, I never imagined she would have to do that. At one point I was wishing for her life to stop. Gradually she became quiet, everything slowed down. Slow and tortuous. Material came out of her mouth and bowels.

Death isn't pretty, it's ugly. I'm angry at her rambling in the last 24–48 hours of her life. It seemed so cruel, so unnecessary. Maybe it meant she was anxious and we should have done something to help that.

Joannie is gone. We were both in the car picking up tickets for the Tucson trip. I went into the pharmacy and came out. She was gasping for breath. I drove through five stop signs to the nearby hospital. The hardest thing to say was do not resuscitate, but I heard Joannie's voice saying, "If you resuscitate me I'll kill you." She died within two hours. I was by her side."

Ben died at 3 AM. I was on the phone to a nursing agency. I heard a commotion in the living room. Ben was trying to get off the couch while E. and a friend were trying to keep him on it. I said he wants to move why are you stopping him. We helped him into a wheelchair, wheeling him to the bedroom. I knew something terrible was happening by his whole demeanor. I called the doctor who pronounced him dead. I would have given my life for him.

George died at 5 AM. Vomiting yesterday, right leg jerking to overwhelming pain, so tremendous that it took him away. He had three grandmal seizures before his death. I'm so glad he didn't have pneumonia or anything.

The suffering he went through is difficult to deal with. Sorrow and anger that he was not rendered rapidly unconscious when he had shortness of breath. But also understood the power/alertness/keen edge of his mind, his smiling as I sang to him a Yiddish love song. We were as one skin.

I wanted it to be over. I wanted her to have no gag reflex, no blink reflex, no movement. It's a lot of crap when people said she was not experiencing anything, how did one know? Even if no memory of it, experienced it, I went crazy when nurses turned her to prevent "painful bed sores" and saying "her vital signs are great, she may live for a long time." I came very near to putting a pillow over her face.

I heard him coughing, then I heard this God-awful noise. I rushed in. He looked as though he'd had a stroke. I called 911. The ambulance took him to a local hospital. They were very kind, respected his wishes not to resuscitate, kept him comfortable, he died quietly.

It was terrible. He was so emaciated, his heart took so long to give out. It was a titanic struggle between him and cancer. He was incontinent during the last 2–3 days, gurgling and drooling from his mouth the last 24 hours, shallow breathing during the last few hours. The last two weeks were very sad. Sad is a better word than horrible. He was not without a family member by his side for the last two weeks.

The image left from witnessing a torturous death leaves a vivid imprint on the family, which is difficult to erase.

Reliving the Suffering Prior to Death

The weariness of the families is evident in the examples below. Involvement with prolonged suffering takes its toll.

Didi's end was painful. Incontinent of urine and feces and pain. It was hard during the last month, giving her pills, narcotics, drugging her out, and yet having to give them because of the pain. It created such ambivalence.

Jamie's silent suffering, mourning, the pain, and the indignity. For him I'm glad it's over. I wouldn't want him to go on like that. When I gave him the injection of morphine before doing his dressing, the needle came out the other side of his skin he was so thin. That destroyed me. He was confused over the week before he died, but talked to me of dying two days before he died. He had never been able to do that before. How I cried, and how he told me not to be sad, his time had come. I was called the morning that he died, his breathing had changed. I got there just in time. I am so lonely.

There is such loneliness in the house. Her presence is still here. The last few months of her life were a living hell. I couldn't bear going back to the hospital, it was torturous for both of us. That final night I hadn't wanted to go back to the hospital but she insisted, she said she was going home and she died that night. It seemed so unreal, so many false alarms, told so many times she was dying, I never thought it would really happen. I hoped the doctors would be wrong. The cordotomy killed her, it relieved her pain just enough but left her so helpless, unable to do anything for herself, a death knell, took everything out of her, nothing left to fight for. She suffered an awful lot. I saw the look in her eyes that evening. She saw what was coming and was eager to embrace it, seeing something beautiful and beckoning to her. I miss her a lot.

What can you say? I hope he's resting comfortably somewhere after all the torture he went through.

The words used to recount what it was like to care for the dying family member speak of both relief and pain.

Bereavement: Conclusion

The themes of bereavement expressed by the families of the deceased cancer patients can all be best understood as modalities of finding a transition. Coping with loss and grief, finding closure from the abyss of uncertainty and moral and intellectual conflict, and finding a way to put their nightmares to bed and to go forward—these are the challenges of the grieving families.

Their words are filled with remembering the actual death and attendant suffering, re-creating their experience into terms that enable them to go forward into life. Sometimes relief is expressed, sometimes guilt, sometimes guilt over the relief, but always the sense of the void and the search for what to do now. Most have faced the most difficult period of their lives and their greatest challenges in the period of giving care to their dying loved ones. They have endured the inevitable loss and void and probably the saddest moments of their lives—the biggest wrenching changes imaginable. From this they must find a transition, a way to bring life back to normalcy, a way to get past these experiences. The statements of bereavement are in many ways a history of what has happened to the patients and the families and what they experienced. The transition to a different future is developed in bereavement.

Conclusion

Patient and family are joined together in a community of suffering, and their words reflect the pain of entering and living in this arduous new territory. For the patient, expressions of despair, being trapped, being afraid, aloneness, vulnerability, and sorrow communicate to others in the world a sense of the nature of the suffering felt. These others most often are family members who have undertaken to care for their loved one and who also suffer greatly. Families faced with the ongoing care of patients with advanced cancer become exhausted and overwhelmed with the burden of daily care and decision making. The witnessing of frequent suffering, loss of mental clarity, and progressive loss of function overwhelms and depletes the families. They are confronted with loss of the life they knew, death, and the need to construct a new way of living. Their statements reveal the depth of their exhaustion and anguish. The level of suffering going on in a home where family members are caring for a dying patient is usually unrecognized because it is rarely recorded. The words of the family members bear witness to intense suffering, sometimes expressed in rage and anger, guilt, defeat, numb acceptance of constant loss, and deterioration.

> It's amazing how one stops reacting to these things. I think he lost his vision this weekend, devastated me, but I adjusted and am ready for the next thing.

The above quotation is typical of the shell-shocked family member straining for equilibrium. This is also the force in the process of bereavement. The process of finding a means of transition from the death of the patient back to a normal life of some sort is the outcome of bereavement. Grieving, adjusting, rationalizing, searching for meaning and purpose all are elements of the process of bereavement. After having gone through one of the biggest challenges possible, the survivors must make sense of their experience and understand it in terms that will allow and assist them in going forward with their lives.

References

1. Cherny, N. I., Coyle, N., & Foley, K. M. Suffering in the advanced cancer patient: A definition and taxonomy. *Journal of Palliative Care, 10,* 57–70.
2. Russell, B. (1945). *The history of western philosophy.* New York: Simon & Shuster.
3. Russell, B. (1948). *Human knowledge: Its scope and limits.* New York: Simon & Shuster.

Part Two

Suffering in Special Contexts

Holding On, Letting Go

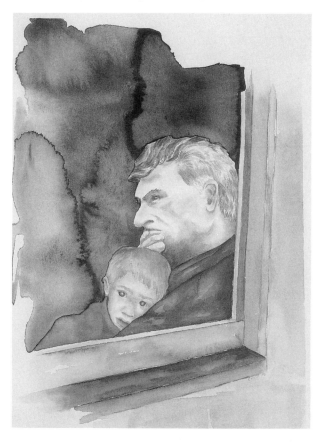

Chapter 3

The Suffering of Children and Families

Barbara S. Shapiro, MD

University of Pennsylvania

In the usual and desirable scheme of events, there is no child without a family, just as there is no baby without a mother (31). Although this is not always the situation, most children, if they are to survive, live within a group of adults who provide some of the functions of a family. The child exists within the family, and because of the family. If the child suffers, so too does the family, and likewise the suffering of the family is echoed within the child.

When serious illness intrudes on any member of the family, some degree of suffering inevitably ensues, as death, the implicit or symbolic threat of death, and separation from cherished others imbue suffering with its unique qualities. The critical question is whether the suffering is overwhelming to the child and the family. The answer is forged by an interplay among the nature of the illness and the symptoms, the functioning of the family, the resources of the child, community support, spiritual beliefs, and the degree to which the health care professionals understand the suffering and provide helpful intercession and support.

The focus of this discussion is on the suffering that children and families endure because of medical illness and medical care, and on the steps that health care professionals can take to minimize (but not eliminate) the suffering. The concept of family will be used in its widest meaning; that is, a group of individuals, not necessarily genetically related, and of almost any conceivable size and composition, whose lives are intimately related functionally and emotionally.

Significance and Impact

Although medically related suffering has been addressed by many authors (7), (23), little has been written about the suffering of children or their families (10), (22), (11). The relative neglect of this crucial area unfortunately parallels the neglect of other areas concerning children and families. For example, many investigators have demonstrated that medically related pain in children *frequently is either not considered or is underestimated,* and is treated even less adequately than pain in adults (24). The manner in which pain is regarded and treated illuminates beliefs and behaviors regarding the larger issues of suffering (25). Cassell says, "Its relief—the relief of all symptoms—is the hallmark of care aimed at the relief of suffering." (7, p. 245). Most health care professionals recognize that children suffer as a result of medical illness and medical care. However, this recognition is often not reflected in priorities nor *translated into actions*.

Societal forces impinge on the awareness of children's suffering. In our society, children are particularly vulnerable to abuse. Furthermore, although our society places a high token value on the welfare of children, this value is not reflected in the spending of tax dollars, the establishment of effective intervention programs, the design of workplaces, or the prestige of people who choose to work with children. The medical arena is comprised of the same social fabric.

Suffering is addressed within human relationships, and the relief of suffering entails time and attentiveness, rather than high technology. If we assume that actual versus token priorities are separable by examining actions, then we see that the actual priorities of medical care are focused on disease and technology rather than on the relief of suffering. Given the social background, we cannot be surprised when medical suffering in children and families is not addressed with the same zeal as are other areas of medical care.

Although the relief of suffering has not held a high priority in the actual practice of medicine, children represent a particularly vulnerable population (21), and since children and their families are inextricably intertwined, the vulnerability extends to the family. The roots of vulnerability are manifold. Children are limited in their physical, cognitive, and communicative abilities, and carry little social power or prestige. Therefore, they are unable to act as their own advocates, and depend on others to do so (25). The extent of their suffering may not be heard or understood by adults, as their verbal communicative abilities are limited. We understand the suffering of others by communication and by empathy, and adults, by repressing or denying memories of their own childhood suffering, may not be empathic to the suffering of children.

When adults do hear and understand the suffering of children, the realization may be painful. One way to deal with this pain is to then minimize the experience. This defense is frequently and clearly seen in medical settings, when adults tell children or themselves that "it does not hurt that much," or when they delete the awareness of the child's pain from their consciousness.

The concept of redemptive suffering runs deep in our society, and adults may rationalize suffering by assuming that it is for the eventual good of the child. The helplessness that adults feel when faced with a child's suffering is uncomfortable, and this discomfort is lessened by denial, minimization, and rationalization. Additionally, since hostility, rage, hatred, and sadism are an integral part of human nature, and since medical care takes place within human interactions, we must assume that these forces may find expression in that care.

The small size of children may lead adults to assume that their emotions, concerns, and fears are also small. However, this is not the case. Emotions such as love, hate, anger, fear, terror, sadness, and jealousy are experienced intensely by children. Differing emotional and cognitive structures influence the texture of emotions, but not the intensity. The limited cognitive understanding of children, along with their inexperience in modulating and understanding their responses may actually sharpen the intensity of their emotions. Children struggle in their own way with the existential concerns of essential aloneness, dependence, autonomy, and fears of annihilation and death that plague adults. They just do not express these concerns through "great" art, literature, philosophy, or creative works of science.

Similarly, children have the capacity to suffer as much as adults, and perhaps more. To assume otherwise is to assume a Pollyanna view of childhood, which perhaps reflects our wish that children did not suffer, or that we did not suffer as children. Children are more likely than adults to be overwhelmed by their suffering, as their coping skills, defenses, and resources are limited. Children suffer differently than adults, just as all individuals suffer differently. Suffering, like pain, is a multifaceted experience, partaking of physical, cognitive, emotional, social, cultural, and spiritual dimensions. Since children differ developmentally from adults in all these spheres, the quality of their suffering is inevitably different.

As for many human experiences and emotions, suffering lies within a four-dimensional framework. One of the dimensions is *intensity*. One can suffer a little and one can suffer a lot. The same child may suffer from severe pain and from unexpressed fears of death, but one of these experiences may be more intense than the other. The second dimension is *quality*. A child who receives treatment for cancer from ages 5 to 10, at which time she dies, most likely suffers differently at the time of diagnosis and when nearing death.

The third dimension is *impact*. We suffer because of a perceived threat to physical, emotional, or social well being and integrity. Up to a certain point, we maintain emotional and social integrity despite the perceived threat. However, at a certain point the perceived threat becomes real, and the person experiences a disintegration of the self.

When this is physical, we call it death. When this is emotional and relational, we call it trauma. Children are vulnerable to overwhelming suffering, or trauma. Similarly a family which is already vulnerable because of its particular composition and function is likely to disintegrate, or undergo trauma, in response to the overwhelming illness or death of a child. However, no matter what the strengths, all individuals and all families have a critical point beyond which suffering becomes traumatizing.

The fourth dimension of suffering is *time*. The longer suffering continues, the more unendurable it becomes, although the ability to endure is of course influenced by the other dimensions and by the resources of the individual, the family, and the system. Also, continuing suffering may erode the very strength that is necessary for endurance, thus contributing to disintegration. Time is particularly important when considering the suffering of children and families. Time is a relative rather than an absolute construct; a short time for an adult may be an eternity for a baby or a young child. Therefore, we, as adults, cannot apply our concepts of duration and endurability to children. Because children suffer so readily in what seem to us to be short times, and because the welfare of children and their families are intertwined, families too can suffer in what seem to be short times.

We can view suffering in families as being both an experience of the individual and an experience of the system. Ordinarily we do not think of systems as suffering. However, since the family system partakes of the experiences of all the individuals, but is in fact not reducible to these experiences, the individual suffering is expressed within a larger sphere, which for want of a better term we can call family suffering. The dimensions of suffering that apply to individuals—intensity, quality, impact, and duration—also apply to families. Similarly, the constituents of individual suffering—physical, emotional, social, cultural, and spiritual—apply to families.

Avoidable and Unavoidable Suffering and the Responsibility of Health Care Professionals

Pain and suffering are integral parts of human existence. However, some suffering is necessary and unavoidable, and some is unnecessary. Within this distinction, we can examine the concept of the redemptive value of suffering, as it applies to children, and the responsibility of the health care professional.

Despite the best efforts of parents, politicians, societies, and health care professionals, much disease and trauma is unavoidable. Similarly, suffering due to medical illness, and to the potentially curative medical treatments and procedures used, is also unavoidable. No matter how supportive and compassionate the medical care, when a child is diagnosed with a disease such as leukemia, the family and the child will suffer with the threat of death. In such situations, although we can provide maximal analgesia and anxiolysis using pharmacologic, cognitive-behavioral, and psychological approaches, procedures such as bone marrow aspirates and lumbar punctures produce anticipatory anxiety and suffering over the possible results. No child would choose to have a bone marrow aspirate. No matter how much the health care professionals seek to cure and save children from death, some children will die, and they and their families will suffer. Such suffering is unavoidable.

Pain, distress, anxiety, and frustration are necessary to growth and development. When these experiences are tolerable and mild, the child does not suffer, and may gain strength as a result of the experience. For example, children fall and hurt themselves when they begin to explore the world. The child who is never hurt in this context is probably not exploring. The parents have the responsibility to make sure that the injury is not severe. If the parental response is appropriate, the child learns to tolerate and recover from minor injuries. Chemotherapy is necessary to cure childhood cancer. Although the medication may produce nausea, vomiting, fatigue, alopecia, and hospitalization because of fever and infection, the attendant suffering is necessary, if and when the chemotherapy is necessary.

If chemotherapy that had no symptomatic side effects was as effective as currently available chemotherapy, administration of the medication with the side effects would be as unthinkable as tripping a toddler so that she learns to tolerate falls and pain. In the treatment of disease and injury, as in the rest of life, when it is possible to reduce or avoid pain, anxiety, and suffering, without producing more suffering in the long run by these efforts, the health care professional must do so. Thus the health care professional is aware of all ways to minimize present and future suffering, and is sometimes forced to weigh present versus future suffering. For example, telling a child and her family that she has a serious and potentially life-threatening illness produces suffering. Talking in euphemisms or lying would decrease the immediate suffering, but with very deleterious long-term effects. However, giving the bad news without going slowly, allowing for hope, and providing privacy and support fulfills the requirement for truth telling, but produces unnecessary suffering. The health care professional is forced to simultaneously assuage and tolerate suffering. This can be a very difficult situation, as compassion and empathy must consistently be tempered with logic and objectivity, in a manner that is helpful for the patient, the family, and the health care team. Very different strengths and reactions must coexist.

When it is not possible to avoid suffering, the health care professional can almost always find ways to help the child and the family tolerate the experience without disintegration. In order for this to happen, the health care professional must be aware of, attentive to, and respectful of the sources of suffering for children and their families. Such attentiveness reduces the essential loneliness of suffering.

Sources of Suffering

Suffering has physical, emotional, cognitive, social, and spiritual components. These components can be heuristically separated, but in actuality are inextricably interrelated. For example, the parents of a sick newborn baby on a ventilator may be sitting immediately at the bedside. If, however, they are unable to hold the baby, the baby will experience the lack of holding in physical terms. Social isolation is emotionally deadly. Physical pain affects emotional well being.

Cultural forces affect all components of suffering. Conditions that produce suffering in one culture may not in another culture. Furthermore, helpful reactions to suffering are shaped by the cultural background of the family. Rarely is it beneficial to challenge cultural beliefs in the course of treating illness or injury, unless the cultural backgrounds or beliefs of the child and family differ, or unless the welfare of the child is in jeopardy. For example, some cultures believe that a person who is dead should not be mentioned, or that one should not talk about death with a dying person. When such beliefs are truly cultural rather than solely defensive, the family can be helped to support the child in its own way. A child is not helped by being in the middle of a cultural disagreement between the parents and the health care professionals.

In illness and trauma, the sources of suffering are often multiple. A baby in a neonatal intensive care unit may experience pain from multiple procedures, overstimulation from lights and noises, lack of restorative sleep, isolation from parents, lack of soothing and loving holding and touch, lack of oral stimulation except for noxious procedures, uncomfortable positions, rapid and jerky handling at unpredictable times, and a variety of other uncomfortable stimuli. A child with cancer could have pain, nausea from chemotherapy, lack of adequate and restorative sleep, separation from parents, worry about death, embarrassment over appearance, and lack understanding of the reasons for multiple procedures and hospitalizations.

The individual contributors to suffering may in and of themselves be large or small. However, the total outcome of suffering is similar to stress; stress can result from a single overwhelming stressor, or from the accumulation of multiple small hassles, or both. Although impending death, with all its suffering for the child and the family, may not be preventable, addressing the multiple smaller sources of suffering can do much toward easing the total burden for the child and the family. Additionally, the mere act of attentiveness to the small details of suffering reassures the child and family that they are not alone in their suffering—and that sense of a committed physician or nurse being with them is perhaps the most powerful force we can wield.

Suffering in Ill or Injured Children

The Need for Comfort

Pain is one of the most common causes of suffering in patients of all ages. Pain related to disease, medical procedures, and trauma in babies and children can be safely and effectively minimized, although not eliminated, by using a combination of pharmacologic, cognitive-behavioral, psychological, and physical interventions (5). Chronic or recurrent pain unrelated to disease or trauma can be more difficult to treat, but the total suffering of the patient can be decreased using a combination of approaches.

Other symptoms also contribute to suffering. These include but are not limited to nausea, vomiting, constipation, fatigue, pruritus, lack of restorative sleep, dry mouth, and dizziness. Children may be unable to communicate these symptoms, so that careful assessment and a high index of suspicion are imperative.

However, these other symptoms, although very unpleasant, usually do not have the symbolic connotations of pain. Pain is experienced by children, adolescents, and adults as a metaphor for illness and death (10). Babies likely experience pain as undifferentiated badness coming from without, no matter what the source of the pain, and children up to the age of 12 (and often older) verbally express their understanding of pain as a punishment for their inner badness and wrongdoing (13). This conception of pain as a punishment may remain in the unconscious, as expressed in the Greek root word for pain, which means penalty or punishment.

Thus, the symbolic qualities add to the intolerable nature of continuing severe pain, as when an experience is construed as punishment for one's badness, and suffering gains a new and tormenting dimension. Alternatively, the child (or adult) who consciously or unconsciously feels that punishment is deserved may not mention the pain to parents or health care professionals.

The Need for Attachment

Social connectedness is a vital requirement for all humans. For children, growth and development are adequate only if and when the needs for attachment are both met and maintained. When the early needs for love and attachment are not met, children starve emotionally and sometimes physically, becoming withdrawn, apathetic, and irritable (27), (4). Babies hospitalized in neonatal intensive care units after birth may never have their needs for attachment met.

Likewise, after an attachment with a parent has been formed, separation can be traumatic, especially if the environment is unfamiliar and full of noxious experiences and overstimulation. Abrupt separation from parents is akin to abandonment in the experience of a young child. A 16-month-old toddler who has surgery and emerges from anesthesia in a recovery room without a familiar person present has no way of knowing that she will be reunited with the parent in a few hours. The terror and disorientation may overwhelm the child's tenuous ability to soothe and comfort herself. Although the parents have not in fact abandoned the child, the child's experience is what we need to consider.

The effect of separation on the child will be determined by age and developmental issues, length of separation, preparation of the child, context, the child's temperament and inner resources, the degree of illness, and the reactions of other adults. Separations that are tolerable in the normal course of events become intolerable when combined with hospitalization, painful procedures, debilitating illness, and lack of other supporting and comforting adults. Children (and adults) who are ill and physically debilitated have fewer emotional resources with which to cope with separation and pain. When we consider that the maintenance of social contact is important in the outcomes of adults with serious illness (6) and for women in labor (18), we realize that for children maintenance of connectedness is even more crucial.

Rarely is it necessary to separate an ill child from her parents, except when the parent is unable to be helpful to the child even with the guidance of health care professionals. Hospitals have progressed from the days when parents were forbidden to stay with their children. However, unnecessary remnants of these practices still persist.

Both the physical and the emotional presence of the parent are necessary to prevent an intolerable sense of loss and lack of protection in the child. Some parents are physically present, but due to their own suffering are unable to provide necessary support to the child. Similarly, parents may feel very close to and supportive of their child, but due to pragmatic concerns be unable to maintain a physical presence. Intervention to help parents with their own emotional concerns and with pragmatic issues is necessary to reduce the suffering of ill children.

Although we typically think of parents as protecting their children, in times of serious illness and stress the reverse sometimes occurs, and children desperately and gallantly try to protect their parents. This act has many roots. Children deeply love their parents, and it is only human to protect that which one loves. The ability to be empathic with others develops early in childhood, as any parent who has had a toddler come and stroke her face at a time of distress can attest. Children sense their parents' distress and grief over their illness, and wish to spare them from this. In addition, children often feel responsible and guilty for causing their parents' grief. If they can protect their parents from the distress, then their own burden of responsibility and guilt will be lessened. Since children may feel that their illness in some way resulted from a previous wrongdoing, the situation becomes very complicated in terms of responsibility and guilt. For example, an adult who is a survivor of childhood cancer relates his thinking at the age of 4 that the cancer was a punishment for his death wishes toward his little brother. Children need the protection of their parents, and worry that if their parents are too overburdened, they will not be able to continue their role as protectors. Children may also be angry at their parents for "allowing" the illness to occur, and then in their conflict over that anger seek to protect the parents.

Usually children are not directly aware of the substance of these worries and guilts, and feel only confused and driven unless they have the opportunity to explore their concerns. This process may be heightened if the parents (and the health care professionals) are indeed too burdened by their own reactions to tolerate the child's feelings.

A clinical example of the protection of the parent is that of a 4-year-old boy with terminal neuroblastoma. He was noted to be consistently lying very still in his bed, not playing or sleeping well. However, the child did not cry, and when asked said he did not hurt at all. His mother knew intellectually that he was dying, but expressed the belief that his tumor was still responding to chemotherapy. She believed he was not playing or moving because he was tired. On careful assessment, when given an outline of a child's body, and asked to color in his pain using colors he had chosen, the patient colored the most severe pain in a pattern that reflected his ultrasound and CT scan—i.e., going down the spine, with twigs radiating into the legs, which presumably were sciatica. As he drew his pain, his mother watched. Initially she appeared surprised and distressed, but then was able to listen and allow him to express his pain.

In retrospect, the child knew from past experience that pain represented disease and caused distress and sorrow in his mother, and he was protecting her from this knowledge and himself from her reaction. The boy was given analgesics for his pain, and was playing the next day. He and his mother were able to continue talking about his pain, and his mother began to accept that he indeed had progressive disease. He died comfortably two weeks later.

Another situation that interferes with the parent's ability to provide comfort and protection for the child is the common practice of asking parents to aid in physically restraining their children during painful or distressing procedures. Under no circumstances should a parent be asked to do this, unless it is for a brief hug to hold the child during a routine procedure such as an immunization or venipuncture. Parents should be with their children during procedures (1), (5), but their role is to comfort, not to force and restrain. Guiding the parents in this role also reduces the suffering of the parents, as they need to comfort and soothe their children. This increases their own sense of control. When parents are forced to restrain their ill children for painful procedures, they may cope by becoming angry at the child for struggling. This response is not helpful for either the child or the parent.

For example, a 3-year-old girl had anxiety-provoking and mildly painful procedures scheduled about every four weeks for a skin condition. The procedures lasted about fifteen minutes. The author observed the child during one of the procedures. The child became frightened and started crying before going into the procedure room. In the procedure room, she was placed in a restraining device, but due to the nature of the procedure her arms had to be free. Her father was asked to hold her arms still, while the nurse held her head.

The child screamed and struggled during the entire procedure. Initially the father was gentle and careful while restraining her. However, after about five minutes, his face became grim and angry appearing. In response to the child's scream, "Let go, let go, you're squeezing me!", he responded by yelling at her, "If you would just stay still I would not have to squeeze you." The situation deteriorated from there.

This is not an unusual situation; parents cannot be expected to be supportive and reassuring while restraining a screaming, struggling, sweating child. The guilt and sorrow over seeing one's child suffer changes into anger at the child; if the child would not struggle so, the situation would not be so difficult.

The primary intervention in this situation was to change the roles and interactions among the physicians, the nurses, the parent, and the child. Additionally, pharmacologic and cognitive-behavioral strategies were suggested.

Children and families fear being alone with their experiences, fears, and concerns. Community support can buttress the family in its struggles. However, especially in extended or serious illnesses, the health care professionals become vital figures in minimizing isolation. The role of physicians and nurses as powerful and beneficent supporters should not be underestimated. Even when the contents of the burden of suffering cannot be altered, the felt presence and caring of the physician or nurse actually decreases suffering. Children over the age of about three may feel this as acutely as adults. A 6-year-old with cancer, who awakens with stomach pain while in the hospital, may be better able to settle and relax after the physician examines her, pronounces that the pain is from the chemotherapy and not from anything dangerous, and tells her and her parents that a medication will be given in just a few minutes to help with the pain. Obviously, the reaction of children to physicians and nurses varies with their past experiences. Some chronically ill children are frightened of white coats and the laying on of hands.

Physicians unwittingly may avoid visiting children who are dying in the hospital. However, the maintenance of daily attentive visits is as important for the children as for the parents. Even though the physician may know that nothing medical is gained by listening to the child's heart and lungs and feeling her pulses, the examination provides an opportunity for touch, and is experienced as a demonstration of caring. Finally, even when a child is comatose, health care professionals must continue to speak as if the child hears and understands every word. This may be the reality, and parents gain solace in the thought that their dying or comatose child may indeed be able to hear them speak or feel their touch. One of the exceptions is when a child is neurologically brain dead, based on careful examination and EEG. In these situations, acting as if the child can hear and understand breeds false hopes in the parents.

The Fear of Death

Fears of annihilation, mutilation, and death are ubiquitous. Even before children cognitively comprehend death, they fear annihilation. For example, babies react with what appears to be terror and then rage to a sudden drop or change in position. After the age of 15 to 18 months, fears of mutilation become significant, and serious illness and medical procedures almost always elicit these fears. Mutilation fears can be very concrete and specific throughout childhood. As they are often unrelated to adult conceptions of physiology and reality, these fears may not be understood or elicited. For example, a 3-year-old child may react to the words "we are going to take your blood" with abject terror, as she visualizes her body as a container filled with blood being drained of all its essential inner contents. The fears of annihilation and mutilation persist in inchoate and often unconscious forms through adult life.

By about age four, children become aware of the more cognitive concept of death, building on their previous experiences of separation and fears of mutilation and annihilation. Children's conceptions of death reflect their cognitive development, and probably do not approach adult form until the school years. Nevertheless, although a 5-year-old may not understand death as we do, she still knows that people and animals die, that death involves separation, that it causes great grief, and that she could die. She may also understand that adults do not like to talk about these things.

Children frequently feel very alone in their fears and fantasies of mutilation and death. Young children are cognitively unable to separate fantasy from reality by themselves, and unexpressed fears become powerful terrors. Because adults are viewed as powerful and knowledgeable authorities, accurate information expressed simply and concretely can do much to allay children's fears and fantasies. However, parents, because of their own fears, may be unable to talk with their children about these matters. The children sense the parents' fears, and keep their thoughts to themselves.

Often health care professionals contribute to this communicative isolation. The professionals have their own fears of death, especially when a child is involved, and may not be able to talk with the children or help the parents to do so. Explicit and implicit collusions among health care professionals and parents to withhold information from children are not uncommon in medical settings. Parents cannot be expected to know how to talk with their children in unusual situations of serious illness. However, health care professionals must be able to intercede.

At the same time, giving a child too much information or forcing a child to talk about subjects that she wishes to avoid can be hurtful. The type of information given must be adjusted to the age and personality of the child. Too little information can inflame fantasies, and too much information, especially if it is not given with an awareness of developmental issues, can inflame fears and shatter defenses. Denial, when used in moderation, is valuable. No one can contemplate their own death or the death of a loved one constantly. Reprieve is necessary.

Children who lie in their hospital beds without diverting activities may be forced into melancholic withdrawal, as their defenses are overwhelmed by contemplation of reality and fantasy. Children must be provided with play and art activities. A hospitalized child can be brought into the hallway or the playroom during the day, so that she is exposed to social interactions. Art therapy, play therapy, video games, taped recordings of stories, and television are useful in the child's room. Metaphors, stories, art work, and imagery help reticent and fearful children work through difficult issues slowly, safely, and at their own pace. Specialized personnel are usually not necessary to provide such interventions, as parents can be guided in providing appropriate activities. Such guidance helps parents feel less helpless and more in control.

The Need for Control

Starting early in the second year of life, all humans require a perception of control over at least some aspects of their environment. The extent of actual control varies with age and situation, but removal of a previously established level of control is felt keenly, and undermines self esteem. We suffer and rage over that which we feel we cannot control. Illness is usually not controllable, and intrudes despite all efforts. In addition, hospitals tend to remove control over personal tasks and decisions from patients and families [10], [22].

Control over life and death is not usually possible, but control over smaller issues can be preserved. However, the preservation of control may require a modification of hospital routines and expectations. The extent of children's control must be appropriate to their age and development. Too much control is alarming; too little is enraging. Children and families can help in planning daily schedules, regulating analgesia [14], [20] and symptom control, keeping track of symptoms, and performing daily hygiene and tasks.

The Need for Visibility

Children are at times treated by health care professionals as if they were invisible. For example, physicians may address the parents and not the child. Physician's rounds may be held in the hallway, within sight of the child and the parents, but without including them in the conversation. Nurses may talk to coworkers at the bedside, ignoring the child. During procedures, physicians and nurses at times deal with their own anxiety by engaging in jokes and banter. Children report outrage over this practice, especially when the conversations are "over their heads," or jokes and innuendoes are made without including the child in producing the humor. The sense of being invisible is deeply disconcerting for individuals of all ages, especially when they are trying to maintain their sense of self-wholeness in the face of serious illness.

The Need for Validation

The lack of validation or a direct contradiction of a child's expressed subjective experiences is a source of considerable anger and confusion. This problem is frequently seen in the assessment of pain, when the child is told that the pain is not as bad as she says, or that it is "in her head." Patients of all ages with chronic pain are often told that the pain is "in your head," and the first part of any effective treatment consists of dealing with their anger and confusion over these statements. The patient knows that the pain is in her body, hears the statement as pejorative (which it often is), and then secretly wonders if maybe she is "crazy." The physician, in making the statement, may be stating her assumption that emotional factors are maintaining or influencing the pain, but is unable to communicate the interplay of emotional factors with pain in a positive manner, and in effect cancels the patient's experience and concerns.

Health care professionals can choose to disagree with patients and families over treatments and interpretations. However, subjective experiences are the property of the person experiencing them. Challenging or contradicting the experience erodes the boundaries between individuals, and makes no sense intellectually, emotionally, or therapeutically. Children are particularly vulnerable to such invalidation, as they tend to question their own sensations and perceptions. Lack of acceptance of inherently subjective phenomena results in either a withdrawn and confused child, or a child who exacerbates her symptoms in an attempt to gain belief.

The Need for Quiet

Overstimulation is often a problem in hospitals. The environments are full of lights, noises, beepers, interruptions, fragments of conversations, disruptions of sleep, unusual odors, large machines, and hospital personnel scurrying in and out of rooms and past bedsides. Humans of all ages require times of quiet and restoration, especially when they are ill. In adults, the overstimulation of the intensive care unit can lead to a transient psychosis. We must consider what the same environment does to babies, who are unable to clearly communicate their inner states.

To avoid suffering or self-fragmentation, babies and children require some sort of reprieve from the onslaught. As in many situations, it is not possible to remove all, or nearly all, the stimulation. However, simple measures such as the introduction of screens, reducing lights at night, quieting voices, reducing speed of movement, and providing predictable times during which the patient is not disturbed for procedures unless there is an emergency can do much toward reducing the total burden of stimulation. For older children and adolescents, the related need for privacy can be respected by knocking at the door and establishing with the child times and places for privacy.

The Search for Meaning

Children seek meaning for their suffering, as do their parents and other adults in their lives. The search for meaning, alloyed with the search for connectedness, provides a way to transcend immediate experience. We may choose to call this process spirituality. For very young children, the search for transcendent meaning may be evident in small everyday rituals. These rituals symbolize and provide a structure for closeness and love, the passage of time, and the rhythms of existence. Older children retain the need for rituals, but also seek other meanings for their experiences. When there is meaning, the burden of suffering and the risk of disintegration decreases (12), (2).

The meaning of illness varies greatly among individuals, families, and cultures. The meaning of illness and suffering may be different for a child and for an adult. However, within families, personal meanings are often communicated, and one family member's understanding will influence other family members. The meaning may be relational (it brought us closer), personal (now I appreciate the important things in life), existential (life is taking the good with the bad), or religious (this is God's will). Respect and understanding for children's and parents' search for meaning helps with that search, and thus helps with suffering.

The Misuse of Behavior

Children's behaviors may be misunderstood, and those behaviors which are easier for the health care professionals and parents to tolerate are encouraged or viewed as adaptive. In reality, the child who does not cry during procedures, is compliant with other regimens, and does not get angry may be suffering greatly. Children who use externalizing defenses tend to be given intervention more readily than children who tend to internalize. The emergence of anger and irritability after a long and debilitating illness is often a sign of recovery. Too often in health care settings, children's behaviors are equated with inner experience. In reality, behavior is a complex amalgam of inner experience, cultural mores, temperament and inherent coping style, learned responses, emotional resources, adult reactions, and degree of debilitation. Behavior tells us how a child copes, not what she is feeling. Many children who suffer do so quietly, but are quite willing to relinquish their burden to a trusted person.

Suffering in Families

Before we discuss the suffering of families, the function of the family must be examined. Families provide many functions for their members. The functions vary depending on ages, inner strengths, and outer circumstances. Although a family can be understood as a system, the individuality of each member should not be lost in the system, although the extent to which the individuality is either prized or subsumed into the system varies among families and cultures. What is helpful for a family in one culture is not necessarily helpful in another culture.

Physical and emotional *protection* of the members is one function of the family. The same actions may result in overprotection for one member of the family, and underprotection for another. The degree to which protection is helpful also varies over time for each person. Families provide and meet needs for *connectedness and continuity*. One hopes that the primary emotion felt within families is love. However, even in the most well-functioning families, a web of complex, ambivalent, and highly changeable emotions exists. The family provides a place where children and adults experience intense love, hate, rage, jealousy, loss, and other emotions, all of which provide connectedness. The well-functioning family provides safety and protection of self and others within this web of emotions. Another function is *communication*, which may be verbal or nonverbal, cognitive, and emotional. Families ensure *survival*. Every member of the family has a pragmatic function, however that function is observed. Even young children help with simple household chores. *Support* is vital to the cohesiveness of a family. Even family members who fight constantly with one another unite in defense when the attack comes from without. Families provide a *trial ground* for activities, interests, and pursuits. A parent considering a career change will usually talk this over with other family members before making a decision. Similarly, children will practice for school performances within the relatively safe arena of home. The family is the *teaching ground* for relationships, ethical values, and spirituality. Even though adults may choose different paths and values than their parents, nevertheless their thoughts and choices are inevitably influenced by the early environment and teaching. Finally, the family is the *model for the larger community*. A child exists first within a dyadic relationship, and then moves into a more complicated system with multiple family members. Many larger group and political processes consist of the same forces—love, hate, jealousy, power, loyalty conflicts—that exist within a family.

All the functions and properties of a family interact, as do family members (even when the interaction is in purposeful avoidance). Additionally, all factors impinging on any individual also impinge on the whole system. One can examine the functions of a family, and see how the serious illness and suffering of a child would affect or possibly erode every one of these functions. The separation of a child from the family for hospitalization is painful for the other members of the family. Siblings, in addition to missing their brother or sister and worrying about his or her welfare, may feel guilty because they previously had wished vehemently for such a possibility. Grandparents have their own special relationships with their grandchildren; these relationships are often disrupted by severe illness. Grandparents may be called upon to act as parents, or may feel excluded from the decision making.

Hospitalization and illness often stretch a family to its limits, with one parent staying at the hospital and caring for the sick child, and the other parent (if there is one) taking on all the burdens of the rest of the family. Emotional energies are taxed, leaving little available to communicate effectively among family members and to provide for regulation of the web of family emotions (10), (22). Sexual relationships between spouses may be disrupted, and generational boundaries blurred. When children are hospitalized for long periods of time, and a parent stays with the child, that parent may begin to consider the hospital as the family. Illness and hospitalization disrupt family rituals. Financial resources may be expended, and work placed in jeopardy because of numerous absences to care for the child, leading to fears of all family members about the survival of the family.

The death of a child is felt by all families to be unnatural. Death and the process of dying leave the family and its members with ever-present scars, even if the open wounds heal. Making reparations and saying goodbyes is necessary but difficult. Parents and siblings usually have guilts—guilts of omission and commission, and guilts that are based in reality as well as in fantasy. These guilts may not need to be addressed directly or explicitly, but somehow each member of the family must come to terms with these feelings. Siblings especially may have a difficult time, as they are often relatively and unavoidably neglected during the illness of the patient, and they are riddled with intense jealousy and guilt.

Children who die live on in the memories of the survivors. If the child dies in pain and anguish, this will be the memory of the family, even if it is never spoken. Therefore, optimal intervention for pain and suffering is crucial, not just for the child as she is dying, but also for the other family members and their memories.

Developmental Considerations

In order to understand and assuage the suffering of children, we must understand their cognitive, emotional, and social development. This discussion focuses particularly on preverbal children, as health care professionals often find it easier to understand the suffering of children who can express themselves verbally.

Babies

The primary need of babies is to be loved and protected. Babies crave and require human contact, expressed by touch as well as by sight, sound, and smell. Physical protection and emotional love are interdependent. If one loves a baby, but has no physical contact, that baby will not feel loved. Babies have no way to understand the reasons for pain. Therefore, all pain, whether inflicted via a lifesaving medical procedure or inflicted as abuse, is equally anguishing (8). For older children and adults, understanding the meaning lying behind pain helps make the difference between bearable and unbearable pain. Such is not true for a baby.

Babies can tolerate short periods of pain and other distress. For example, immunizations cause pain and distress, but cannot be thought of as causing suffering. Suffering in a baby occurs when an event exceeds the capacity of the baby to relatively quickly reintegrate and settle, given adequate comforting. Taking routine immunizations as an example, if babies are held, rocked, and fed after the procedure, they usually calm within 10 or 15 minutes. However, if the pain and distress should continue, the baby's immediate terror and rage, as expressed by crying, eventually subsides, and the baby becomes irritable, restless, apathetic, or withdrawn. After a certain point, babies no longer respond readily to soothing intervention, and are in a state of disintegration.

Unfortunately, babies' responses to overwhelming suffering may not elicit the necessary responses from health care professionals and other adults. As babies disintegrate, they gradually stop crying and exhibiting other signals of distress. This leads adults to conclude that the baby is adapting and coping. Babies may lapse into sleep not because they have dealt with the experience, but as a way of escaping an intolerable situation or intolerable emotions. This leads to less concern and comforting, which further perpetuates the cycle.

An example is that of a baby who has been chronically and painfully abused physically. Such babies often cry little in response to events such as venipunctures and intramuscular injections—a very different response from the baby who does not expect pain to be a part of life. Health care professionals who are not familiar with the behavior of abused children may mistakenly interpret the behavior as being due to a calm temperament (which is possible, but not the only explanation).

Since babies are not verbal, traumatic experiences are not later communicated verbally to parents or other adults. However, data support the retention of nonverbal memories, which later permeate social interactions and intrapsychic events, and may appear in dreams, nonverbal memory fragments, or play (19), (30), (26), (3), (16), (28), (17). Since the nonverbal communication of previous trauma is often not understood by adults, this leads to the common misconception that experiences that are not (verbally) remembered and communicated are of no or little significance. The lack of access to the experience leads to an underestimation of the degree of suffering of babies and of the impact on future structure.

The parents also suffer when a baby suffers. Few parents are able to watch their baby experience pain without feeling anguish themselves. Even witnessing an immunization can be difficult for parents, although most are able to deal with their reactions by remembering the consequences of not having the immunization. We want parents to experience distress themselves at the thought of their baby's distress. A lack of response in a parent may be an indication of inadequate empathy and bonding. Loving parents also want to be with their babies, and to hold their babies. Separation may be as difficult for a parent, albeit experienced in a different manner, as for a baby. Even the hospitalization of a baby for a few days, although routine for a health care professional, can evoke anguish in the parents. Likewise, the inability to touch a very ill baby can be tormenting for the parent and grandparent. Health care professionals whose babies become ill and require hospitalization or an unusual procedure are often surprised by the vehemence of their reactions when they see their baby undergo the same procedure that they themselves may have performed with little thought on many other babies.

Toddlers

Toddlers have some verbal skills, and can understand simple directions and reassurances. They are acutely attuned to the responses of the parents to guide their own responses, and are beginning to understand that people who go away do come back. They intensely desire control and autonomy, and are fearful of separation. Their sense of time, like babies', is very different than that of an adolescent or adult, and a short period of continued pain, distress, or separation evokes disintegration, manifested as irritability or apathy. Toddlers have no conception of death, but they do fear mutilation, as anyone who has watched a toddler's response to a scrape or cut can attest. However, these fears can be assuaged with familiar rituals, such as the loving application of a band-aid. Toddlers generally value rituals—the rituals of bedtime routines, accompanying their parents to predictable places, being given particular food for meals. Interruption of these routines can be very disturbing, as it invokes the fears of separation and loss of control.

      Thus the circumstances of illness and hospitalization are sources of suffering for toddlers. They need their parents as much as babies, although a transitional object such as a blanket or stuffed toy may suffice for a while. Although rituals cannot be completely maintained as the context and environment are changed, part of the ritual may bolster the toddler's sense of continuity and security. Parents should be allowed and encouraged to be present at all possible times. Because the toddler reacts to the parent's response, parents may benefit from guidance. For example, during a procedure a parent can sit by a toddler's head, talking softly, stroking her cheek, telling simple favorite stories.

Preschool Children

Preschoolers understand simple explanations, and benefit from preparation for potentially distressing events. In addition, they are beginning to formulate their own explanations for events. These explanations revolve around themselves, and preschoolers often assume that distressing events are punishment for their actions. They are able to accept and respond to other explanations. Preschoolers are developing a sense of time, and can tolerate distress for longer than younger children. However, their limits are still much less than for adolescents and adults.

Preschoolers have also absorbed the cultural mores of the parents, and this may alter their willingness to communicate pain and suffering. For example, a 3-year-old child from Vietnam was hospitalized for a serious injury of her leg, which was assumed to be very painful. The health care professionals gave her morphine, but were unable to completely assess her response, as she and her parents spoke no English. The child was lying quietly, not crying or moaning, but the health care professionals arranged for an interpreter. The interpreter ascertained that the child's pain was indeed well controlled, but that she had severe pruritis from the morphine. However, her parents had told her not to scratch, and so she did not. In many other cultures, such obedience to the parents' commands would not be observed.

School-Aged Children

School-aged children are able to understand some consequences, and to have a more formed conception of the future. Rituals continue to be important, but can be varied more than for the younger child. The school-aged child seeks meaningful explanations, and such explanations are often helpful. The school-aged child is often very aware of emotionally regressing during serious illness, and may feel ashamed of the regression.

Adolescents

Adolescence is a stormy time, during which a child grows into an adult sexually, cognitively, emotionally, socially, and spiritually. The changing body habitus, along with growing social awareness and awareness of sexuality, make body changes due to illness very difficult to tolerate.

The school-aged child may tolerate alopecia from chemotherapy in a much more sanguine fashion than the adolescent.

Loss of control and independence are particularly difficult for adolescents, who are already struggling with separation, individuation, and autonomy. Adolescents must be part of the medical decision making, although the decisions cannot be theirs alone. Like school-aged children, adolescents regress during illness, and may benefit from reassurance that bringing a stuffed animal to the hospital is perfectly fine. Continued or profound regression is a sign of trouble. The ill adolescent may be very troubled by existential concerns. Because the adolescent is establishing her independence from the parents, she may need, far more than younger children, to be able to confide in someone outside the family, such as a family friend, favorite teacher, or guidance counselor. Ill adolescents may feel socially isolated, and support groups can help even reticent and shy youngsters to express their concerns.

Conclusions

Children suffer as much as, albeit differently than, adults. Health care professionals who care for children carry the responsibility to assuage that suffering as much as possible. In order to do so, the professionals must be aware of the multiple sources of suffering for children and families, and of how they may contribute to that suffering. This requires a concerted and continued effort, as the easiest way to deal with the suffering of children is to minimize or not notice. Also, health care institutions are organized around the roles of the health care professionals, and not around the comfort and emotional well-being of the patients. Within such environments, individuals may become discouraged, and feel that they can do little. However, such is not the case. Small acts can make a large difference in the total burden of suffering. The easing of a few parts makes the whole more tolerable. An individual's concern and presence imbues patients and families with the sense of not being alone.

In order to effectively help children and their families, health care professionals must deal with their own suffering. It is not easy to watch a child suffer or die, and health care professionals may protect themselves in ways that are not helpful to themselves or to their work. They may become desensitized or "burnt out" and not recognize or heed the suffering of others. The suffering may be denied in a futile quest to prolong life at all costs. Anger at the situation may be projected onto other patients or families, or one's own self, family, or coworkers.

It is inevitable that these protections against unspeakable loss will affect all of us at various times in our careers. However, we can do much to help one another by sharing our distress and conflicts with other health care professionals. It is when we struggle with our anguish by ourselves that we run the greatest risk of engaging in behavior hurtful to ourselves and others.

I would like to recount a dream I had as a third-year pediatric resident. This dream delineates the suffering of health care professionals on several levels. The dream occurred during a brief sleep while "on call" for the oncology service.

> I was giving chemotherapy to a 9-year-old boy with cancer. (He was the same age as one of my own children.) After I gave him the chemotherapy through his IV, he turned into a tiger. I was horrified at what I had done. The tiger ran from the room, and I ran after him, but could not catch him.

> He ran to the River Styx, jumped in, and began to swim across the river. I looked at the water, which was full of flotsam and jetsam. I did not want to jump into the water, so I looked for Charon with his boat, but Charon was nowhere to be seen. In desperation, I jumped into the water and swam after the tiger, for someone had to rescue him.

At that point, my dream was interrupted by a nurse calling to tell me it was time to give chemotherapy to one of the patients. I slammed the phone down without answering, but then as I emerged further from sleep realized what had happened and walked to the nurse's station.

Since this behavior was uncharacteristic of me, after I administered the chemotherapy I told the nurses my dream. One of the nurses, a warm and supportive woman, later gave me a picture of a tiger, which I keep to this day in my office.

References

1. Bauchner, H. (1991). Commentaries: Procedures, pain, and parents. *Pediatric* 87, 563–565.
2. Bettelheim, B. (1952). Surviving and other essays. New York: First Vintage Books.
3. Bolby, J. (1955). Child care and the growth of love. New York: Pelican Books.

4. Bowlby, J. (1988). A secure base: Parent-child attachment and healthy human development. New York: Basic Books.
5. Carr, D. B., & Jacox, A. K. (1992). Acute pain management: Operative or medical procedures and trauma. Washington, D.C.: U.S. Department of Health and Human Services, Public Health Service, Agency for Health Care Policy and Research.
6. Case, R. B., Moss, A. J., Case, N., et al. (1992). Living alone after myocardial infarction: Impact on progress. *JAMA, 267,* 515–519.
7. Cassell, E. J. (1991). The nature of suffering and the goals of medicine. New York: Oxford University Press.
8. Despert, J. L. (1975). The inner voices of children. New York: Simon & Schuster.
9. Famularo, R., Kinscherff, R., & Fenton, T. (1990). Symptom differences in acute and chronic presentation of childhood Post-Traumatic Stress Disorder. *Child Abuse and Neglect, 14,* 439–444.
10. Ferrell, B. R., Rhiner, M., Shapiro, B. S., & Dierkes, M. (In press). The experience of pediatric cancer pain, Part I: Impact of pain on the family. *Journal of Pediatric Nursing.*
11. Foley, G. V., & Whitan, E. H. (1990). Care of the child dying of cancer: Part I. *CA-A Cancer Journal, 40,* 327–354.
12. Frankl, V. E. (1946). Man's search for meaning. New York: Washington Square Press.
13. Gaffney, A., & Dunne, E. A. (1987). Children's understanding of the causality of pain. *Pain, 29,* 91–104.
14. Gaukroger, P. B. (1993). Patient-controlled analgesia in children. In N. L. Schecter, C. B. Berde, & M. Yaster (Eds.), *Pain in infants, children, and adolescents.* Baltimore: Williams and Wilkins.
15. Geoffrey, A., & Dunne, E. A. (1987). Children's understanding of the causality of pain. *Pain 29,* 91–100.
16. Goldson, E. (1991). The affective and cognitive sequelae of child maltreatment. *Pediatric Clinics of North America, 38,* 1481–1496.
17. Green, A. H. (1985). Children traumatized by physical abuse. In S. Eth & R. S. Pynoos (Eds.), Post-traumatic stress disorder in children. *American Psychiatric Press, 7,* 135–154.
18. Kennell, J., Klaus, M., McGrath, S., Robertson, S., Hinkley, C. (1991). Continuous emotional support during labor in a U.S. hospital. *JAMA, 265,* 2197–2201.
19. Kramer, S. (1990). Residues of incest. In H. W. Levine, *Adult analysis and childhood sexual abuse.* Hillsdale, NJ: The Analytic Press.
20. Litman, R., & Shapiro, B. (1992). Oral PCA in adolescents. *Journal of Pain and Symptom Management, 7,* 78–81.
21. Nir, Y. (1985). Post-Traumatic Stress Disorder in children with cancer. In S. Eth & R. S. Pynoos (Eds.), Post Traumatic Stress Disorder in children. *American Psychiatric Press, 6,* 123–132.
22. Rhiner, M., Ferrell, B., Shapiro, B. S., & Dierkes, M. (In press). The experience of pediatric cancer pain, Part II: Management of pain. *Journal of Pediatric Nursing.*
23. Scarry, E. (1985). The body in pain: The making and unmaking of the world. Oxford, England: Oxford University Press.
24. Schechter, N. L., Berde, C. B., & Yaster, M. (1993). Pain in infants, children, and adolescents: An overview. In N. L. Schechter, C. B. Berde, & M. Yaster (Eds.), *Pain in infants, children, and adolescents.* Baltimore: Williams and Wilkins.

25. Shapiro, B. S., & Ferrell, B. R. (1992). Pain in children and the frail elderly: Similarities and implications. In R. Payne, R. (Ed.), *APS Bulletin: Innovations in Practice.*
26. Shengold, L. (1989). Soul murder: The effects of childhood abuse and deprivation. New Haven: Ballantine Books.
27. Spitz, R. A. (1945). Hospitalism: An inquiry into the genesis of psychiatric conditions in early childhood. The Psychoanalytic Study of the Child. New York: International Universities Press.
28. Steele, B. F. (1983). The effect of abuse and neglect on psychological development. In J. D. Call, E. Galenson, & R. L. Tyson (Eds.), *Frontiers of infant psychiatry.* New York: Basic Books, Inc.
29. Stein, H. F. (1990). American medicine as culture. Westview Press, Ltd.
30. Terr, L. (1990). Too scared to cry: Psychic trauma in childhood. New York: Harper & Row.
31. Winnicott, D. W. (1964). Further thoughts on babies as persons. In *The child, the family, and the outside world.* New York: Penguin Books.

Chapter 4

HIV/AIDS and Suffering

See, I've known that for years. I'm not going to die that way. I know, there's going to be some pain, there's going to be discomfort, but I'm not going to suffer. I mean, I just don't suffer well. So I'm not going to.

Jake, Person with AIDS
Died July 4, 1994

Judith M. Saunders, RN, DNSc, FAAN

City of Hope National Medical Center

Introduction

AIDS[1] is an illness associated with suffering. Yet many people with HIV/AIDS speak of triumphs and positive encounters more than suffering and distress (14). Suffering and distress are important dimensions of experiences that people with HIV/AIDS have during their illness, but suffering is one aspect that remains private more than public, unsaid more than said. Why do people with HIV/AIDS remain so silent about suffering? Suffering in silence may not be unique to HIV/AIDS, but may be part of the nature of suffering for people with many illnesses. In one conference on HIV/AIDS in the mid 1980s, a panel of men and women with HIV/AIDS voiced two major messages. The first message was: they had survived having HIV/AIDS so far, were still alive, and wanted the health care indusry to focus more on resources they needed to live quality lives. The second message was: they were not victims; rather they were persons with an illness who focused on staying alive and healthy. The second message heralded a movement to discredit the terminology "victim of HIV/AIDS" and replace it with "person with HIV/AIDS," or PWA. The term, "victim," evoked images of passivity and helplessness, while this deadly disease required people to actively engage in finding ways for infected people to maintain optimal health, become knowledgeable, and resist disease progression (19). Somehow, the terms "victim" and "suffering" seemed inextricably intertwined at this conference. Panel members minimized their suffering experience, like Chad[2] (see Table 4–1) who said, "given all the degrees of suffering, I'm sort of embarrassed to feel like what I've had is suffering, but of course I've suffered."

People generally recognize suffering when discussed by others, and usually can identify their own suffering. On the other hand, HIV/AIDS is perceived as a mysterious illness to people lacking personal experience with someone having HIV/AIDS. Paradoxically, more already is known about HIV/AIDS scientifically than is known about the concept of suffering. What we know about suffering is largely common knowl-

---

[1]AIDS is the endstage of the spectrum of HIV disease. In this chapter, this total spectrum is characterized by using HIV/AIDS. Suffering occurs throughout the course of HIV disease, not only at its end stage. HIV is the abbreviation for Human Immunodeficiency Virus; AIDS is the abbreviation for Acquired Immunodeficiency Disease Syndrome.

[2]Names of all study participants have been changed to protect their anonymity.

TABLE 4–1 Description of Study Participants

Name	Brief Description of Study Participant
Chad	Chad is in his 40s. He is a Caucasian male who became infected through sexual contact with men who were infected. He was an architect before his illness forced him to retire. He has been infected since 1980.
Hillary	Hillary is in her late 40s. She is Asian-Pacific who was born outside the USA, and immigrated to USA 27 years ago. She probably contracted HIV/AIDS through an occupational exposure while working as a laboratory technician. She is recently divorced, and has returned to school to learn a new occupation. She learned of HIV infection in 1991.
Fred*	Fred is in his 40s. He is a Caucasian who contracted HIV/AIDS by having sex with men who were infected. He was an office manager before he was unable to work, but his heart was in music, singing, and dancing. He learned he was infected in 1986.
Miguel	Miguel is in his late 20s. He is Latino who (intentionally) contracted HIV+ from sexual contact with infected males. He learned he was HIV+ in 1991. Does not have AIDS.
Jake*	Jake is in his 40s. He is a Caucasian who contracted HIV+ from sexual contact with infected males. Has been HIV+ since 1983.
Marie	Marie is in her 50s. She is Caucasian. She contracted HIV+ from a blood transfusion while being treated for aplastic anemia. She is in her second marriage, has three children from her first marriage, and is a grandmother. She learned she was HIV+ in 1992.
Doug	Doug is in his 30s. He is Asian-Pacific, born in USA. He contracted HIV+ from sexual contact with infected males. He is HIV+, but does not have AIDS. He learned he was HIV+ in 1989.
Jimmy**	Jimmy is in his 30s. He is both Latino and American-Indian. He contracted HIV+ from sexual contact with infected males or from sharing needles. He continues to use drugs.

*Died summer of 1994
**Died spring of 1995

edge. Only recently have efforts have been made toward understanding suffering conceptually.

This chapter has drawn on the literature, the author's clinical experience, and interviews with people with HIV/AIDS who discuss their experiences of suffering. (See Box 4–1 for a summary of this research.) The findings from these interviews illustrate the chapter. In addition to the definition and concept of suffering, this chapter also discusses features that make individuals affected by HIV/AIDS especially vulnerable to suffering. The chapter ends with discussions of relief of suffering as well as barriers to relief.

Several assumptions have guided the discussions in this chapter: (1) suffering is a personal, subjective experience; (2) suffering is a multidimensional concept with causes (domains), degrees of intensity, and consequences; (3) people who experience suffering know the experience as suffering and can articulate features of their experiences; and (4) illnesses, such as cancer and HIV/AIDS, can evoke suffering.

Suffering as a Concept

Definition

A single definition of suffering has not gained acceptance, and existing definitions that have emerged have been critiqued as unsatisfactory (2). Webster's dictionary (27, p. 2284) defines *suffering* as "the endurance or submission to affliction, pain, loss"; and the verb, *to suffer* as "to submit or be forced to endure the infliction, imposition, or penalty of" and "to go or pass through (as harm or loss)." These definitions imply the following highlights:

1. Suffering is temporal in nature;
2. Suffering can be voluntary or involuntary;
3. Suffering is not a property, rather it is an experience;
4. The person is actively engaged in the experience and exhibits some movement or progress through it;
5. Suffering is an experience triggered by affliction, pain, loss or penalty; and
6. Suffering is located within the person.

Box 4–1   Self-Care, Nursing, and HIV Disease

Purpose:

The overall purpose of the longitudinal, qualitative study (NR00033) was to understand self-care with HIV disease as it is experienced over time and across disease intensity. A smaller study, reported in this chapter, was developed with the specific aim of understanding suffering related to HIV disease as it is experienced by HIV+ men and women. Selected individuals already participating in the longitudinal study were asked if they would be willing to have one of our ongoing interviews focus on their suffering experiences they associated with HIV/AIDS. Study participants were selected only from those who were HIV positive. All study participants who were asked to be interviewed about suffering agreed. The investigator selected study participants to attain a heterogeneous sub-sample by gender, race/ethnicity and degree of illness (HIV positive asymptomatic to AIDS).

Method:

The larger qualitative study (NR00033) of self-care and HIV/AIDS has used unstructured interviews that are tape-recorded and transcribed for better access for analysis. Repeated interviews have been conducted with study participants, and their supportive others, during the three and one half years of this five-year, longitudinal study. The smaller study that focused on suffering and HIV/AIDS included ten interviews with a sub-sample of eight study participants. The question that guided the study on suffering was, "Looking back since you became HIV positive, think of a time that involved suffering for you. Tell me about that experience." All participants in the study on suffering were already participating in the self-care and HIV study. Standard methods of content analysis were used to analyze the data, and to identify common themes. A theme is defined as a common meaning of the interviews, or a meaning that has captured the point of the discussion of suffering among several, if not all, of the study participants. The computer program, Martin, was used to facilitate analysis.

Findings:

The following themes emerged from the study on suffering and HIV/AIDS: Absorbing the impact of learning I have HIV/AIDS; Living with daily stressors and symptoms; Having ties to others as a source of suffering; Facing personal death; Confronting barriers to relief of suffering; Relieving my own suffering; and Receiving help from others.

Funded by the National Institute of Nursing Research (NR00033) Judith M. Saunders, RN, DNSc, FAAN. Principal Investigator

Despite the highlights implied in Webster's definitions of *suffering* and *to suffer*, the concept of suffering remains confusing. Suffering is linked most often with pain, yet this relationship remains cloudy. Spross (21) has emphasized that pain may exist without suffering, just as suffering may exist without pain. Travelbee (23) differentiated physical pain from mental distress and suggested that they combined to form suffering. Lindholm and Eriksson (12) asked patients and nurses to describe suffering and concluded that suffering was neither a feeling nor pain. Kahn and Steeves (11) said that physical pain became suffering when the pain was interpreted by the person as a menace to his/her integrity. Suffering and pain are phenomenologically distinct. Suffering seems to be a concept that is broader than pain: it can include, but is not limited to pain (3), (11), (21).

Suffering is a personal experience, not an external event. Cassell (3) identified many dimensions of personhood that may give rise to the personal experience of suffering, such as a person's role (parent, spouse, nurse, etc.); interpersonal ties; personality and character; memories of one's past; life experiences and their personal meanings; and cultural background. In addition, Cassell (3) identified a person's characteristics that also are important to their potential for personal suffering. These included such qualities as being a political being, doing things, having a secret (private) life, perceiving a future, functioning with various levels of awareness, having routines and regular behaviors, having a physical body and having a spiritual life (i.e., a transcendental dimension). In addition, people develop values that guide their actions; when their actions contradict their values, then they are not in harmony with themselves. This lack of harmony within the self is pivotal to suffering (2), (16). Watson (26) did not use the word "suffering" in portraying illness as disharmony in one's inner self, but her portrayal of illness was consistent with suffering (2). Suffering can arise when the person experiences internal disharmony from any of her/his characteristics or qualities. Suffering can only result if the lack of harmony within the person is bound to a meaningful dimension of one's personhood. How dimensions of personhood can be meaningful and elicit suffering can be clarified by examining the domains of suffering.

Domains of Suffering

Rawlinson (16, pp. 43–50) identified a typology of causes of suffering in four domains: in body, in interpersonal relationships, in the will, and in coherence of the self (unity). Each domain will be summarized and illustrated with experiences of people affected by HIV/AIDS who participated in a study on self-care and HIV/AIDS (see Box 4–1).

Our *bodies* are the homes in which we live and provide us access to the world. We use our bodies to achieve our purposes and maintain our autonomy; suffering arises where a rupture occurs within the person between limits imposed by his/her bodily condition and important purposes. For example, for months, Jake had requested treatment for Kaposi sarcoma (KS) lesions, and the physicians had refused. Then he arrived for a routine appointment a week before a long-awaited trip, and physicians announced they were going to start treatments that day. He asked if treatment could be delayed until he returned, since he already had too many preparations to make and limited time, energy, and resources to cope with unplanned changes in his schedule. Jake said:

> That's the point. I don't have a whole lot of energy to deal with too many variables, and if there's going to be changes, I have to have enough energy to deal with it. So as much as possible I do have control. Especially being as alone as I am, I have to ensure that I spend as little energy on these peripheral things as possible.

Jake's physical distress and his desire for relief and treatment to reverse the KS conflicted with his plans—a trip to the International AIDS Conference where he would learn more and meet others who would provide support to him.

Another example of how body is primary to maintaining personal purpose and autonomy came from Fred. Fred's response was clear and immediate when I asked him to identify and tell me about a time during his HIV/AIDS that he had experienced suffering, ". . . and then he tells me that I have CMV[3] retinitis. That hit me like a ton of bricks." Fred explained that CMV retinitis was one of the first diseases of HIV/AIDS he had heard about, and when he heard about it, everyone who contracted it went blind in six months. Fred highlighted a little of why this mattered so much:

> Yeah, because I wander around here [in his apartment] at night in the dark anyway all the time. Then there, well, I mean if I were

---

[3]Cytomegalovirus. When CMV infection invades the retina, blindness can result, although major advances have been made in treating this disorder.

blind I wouldn't be able to see the light, the street light out in the
alley. It always sort of looks like pale moonlight. It's romantic
without anybody you'd be romantic with, but it would mean that
I probably couldn't play piano again because I can't play without
reading sheet music. Books have to go too. I'd have to learn
Braille.

Both Fred and Jake illustrate the importance of their bodies both
in maintaining personal autonomy and in achieving purposes that
are important. Loss of function as well as pain and other physical
problems lead to suffering by limiting what the body can now do;
such body limitations, in turn, limit achievement and restrict
autonomy.

The second domain, *interactions with others*, is important because it is through these interactions that individuals differentiate their
own possibilities, and take stands on which of those possibilities will
become a part of their own identities. These stands are revealed largely
through the roles that we play with others. When a best friend who
was our greatest critic and supporter dies, we must find other access
to important critique and support, such as incorporating that role into
our own function and/or finding others. As other people are lost to us,
we must recast roles that we play and renew our self-differentiation.
In this manner, losing others also often means a rift within ourselves.
Doug reflected on the changes in Harry's younger brother, Arthur, as
Arthur assumed more and more responsibility during Harry's terminal
illness and death:

> It was really interesting to watch Arthur because I was introduced
> to him about 3 or 4 years ago as Harry's little brother. We met at
> a movie theater and he was Harry's little brother—this sort of very
> silent, meek boy. Through the whole process of becoming Harry's
> executor of his will and standing by him and taking care of him,
> he's very much become a man. It was very interesting to watch
> the process.

Arthur grieved the loss of his brother who was a role model and
friend. In having to be in charge, he had to give up some of his
dependent role and assume more authority and responsibility. His grief
and his role changes both contributed to his suffering.

The third domain, *the will*, shows itself by forging an individual
life history, producing work and accomplishments, and regulating itself
by principles. Miguel illustrated how reviewing his life history helped

him identify a major source of suffering that needed to be reworked if he were going to move beyond the suffering in his life. This source of suffering for Miguel was his lack of resolution of his relationship with his father, and he needed to resolve those issues in order to free himself from a painful past so he could forge ahead with his life. Miguel reported that he realized that he "could no longer tolerate the person I believed I had become or was becoming as a result of my father's abuse, his abandonment of me and my family, and the lack of paternal relationship that developed." To remedy this situation, Miguel struggled a long time to forgive himself and his father. His father was very ill, and it was important for Miguel to resolve this conflict with his father, so he drove to Texas to talk with his father. He later recalled that conversation with him:

> I said I'm here to say goodbye to you [father] because we're not going to see each other again, and I want to put closure to my relationship with you. I want you to know that it's okay. It's okay for you to go [die] when you are ready and that it's fine with me. I've already forgiven myself for whatever I might have done to myself and I'm here to forgive you and to ask you to forgive me before you die. I said, from the bottom of my heart I ask you to forgive me for whatever I might have done, and I just want you to accept my love instead. He said he understood.

Miguel's father died two weeks later. Miguel's reflection on his life history and subsequent reworking of his relationship with his father helped him transcend his suffering. As contradictions emerge in any dimension of the will—life history, accomplishment, and morality or principles—some degree of disharmony within ourselves will appear.

The final domain, *coherence of the self (unity)*, refers to how the individual struggles with and determines purpose and meaning in life. Jake summarized his perspective that his approach is not only central to his experience but also provides meaning and a sense of unity:

> We are ultimately fulfilling our destiny and service to God as we have seen fit. Whether we do it or not has different consequences, and death is not a consequence of life—it's the natural process and how I approach that is how I will experience it. My goal is to be at peace with that, no matter what, and to learn to accept fate or destiny, whatever it is, and I don't even have to know what it is. That's the best I can do.

Key elements in Jake's coherence, or unity, include service to God; his approach to experience and not the experience itself; and acceptance of his fate (life as it presents itself). Jake was active and autonomous in his living with HIV/AIDS; he fought illness progression, confronted doctors when necessary and accepted what he believed were inevitable and unchangeable situations.

Rawlinson (16, p. 49) specifies how suffering emerges, "in each of these orders of meaning, suffering erupts as a rupture within the subject himself, a rupture between his situation and those *ends* that he takes as his own." In speaking of this internal rupture, Jimmy voiced extreme pain:

> I've been drinking wine and I get crazy and I've been fighting with my mom for nothing because I'm in a stupor. I felt awful about it the next day. I didn't want to wake up anymore. I was so stupid. I'm always telling her I hate her in my drunken rages. I scare her and I guess it's like living with a loaded gun. I don't want it to go on. I want to stop everything. I want to stop living. All my guilt. All of the guilt because I treat my mom like shit.

Jimmy has consistently used drugs for years. Sober, he is thoughtful, considerate, and a loving son. Being a loving son is an important end to Jimmy, but he is often at odds with himself—i.e., with the end of being a good son. He has absolutely no strategies to resist drugs and alcohol when they are available. Once suffering emerges, it's intensity may vary.

Intensity of Suffering

Even the simple phrase, "I never suffered so badly in my life," points to the possibility that suffering varies in intensity from one episode to another. Travelbee (23) described suffering as varying in intensity, duration, and depth. Suffering's intensity may not match the objective dimensions of the situations that prompt the internal rupture of harmony that the person will experience as suffering. Instead, the degree of suffering depends on the meaning that the person gives to the situation (3), (22), (23), (25). For example, Hillary spoke of how she suffered from flea bites—certainly a minor inconvenience for most people. She described the flea bites:

> It was so awful. It's painful. This big one especially. They were painful and very itchy. So I suffer from these two episodes of flea

bites. It's been two years since I came back from [the Orient] and the hyper-pigmentation still didn't go away.

For Hillary, pain and itchiness were only part of the suffering and discomfort. Hillary is a very private person who believes that having HIV/AIDS is regarded as both shameful and as a death sentence. The hyper-pigmented areas from the flea bites reveal her problems to others, provoke questions, and threaten to invade her privacy. All these facets combined to enhance her suffering.

For suffering to occur, the individual must perceive the situation as distressing, although the judgment of distress may occur after the immediate situation is over. Travelbee (23, p. 62) included simple transitory discomfort as the lowest range of suffering. She (23, pp. 62–63) also discussed a despairful not-caring that was intense or prolonged with a potential of progressing, and which should be considered an interpersonal emergency. Travelbee (23, p. 63) described the terminal phase of apathetic indifference as the most extreme suffering, which existed beyond despairful not-caring. Miguel identified one depression as a time of suffering, and his experience included a range of intensity. He said:

> And there's different levels of depression. There was when I was able to work and this happened I was still very depressed all the time. And there were times where the depression was so bad that I didn't even want to brush my teeth.

He also described a time in the depression when he was beyond feeling, and just experienced a sense of numbness:

> . . . all that time I was in pain. I did not feel it because I was so depressed, but I was in pain. It was just a numbness. And it is a type of pain that is not really physical that you don't really feel, but you're just in a complete state of hurt.

Suffering is neither a state nor is it associated with a specific level of intensity. An individual's intensity of suffering can vary within the same experience. Suffering may also vary in intensity from one situation to another. Many types of situations can evoke suffering, and HIV/AIDS has several features that increase the person's vulnerability to suffering.

Features of HIV/AIDS That Enhance Suffering

Vasse, a French author (cited in (2)[4]) identified illness, injustice, accident, or death as sources of suffering. Because suffering is a personal experience, individuals will respond differently to situations such as illness. Still, some illnesses are more likely to evoke suffering than others, despite personal response differences. In part, illnesses have variable potential to evoke suffering because of their nature, such as a tendency to cause death, affect children, cause deformity, or interrupt a career. Silverman (20) pointed out that major diseases, such as HIV/AIDS, have problems not only of the disease itself, but also society's reaction to it. In addition to society's negative and judgmental responses to HIV/AIDS, features of the illness, such as chronicity, contagiousness, incurability, and high fatality, enhance potential for suffering.

Society's Reaction to HIV/AIDS

HIV/AIDS has joined other major diseases (e.g., plague or cancer) that have evoked society's reactions of initial denial, then anxiety and hysteria, followed by a search for a scapegoat (20). Society's negative reactions are disclosed by individual actions, as well as in formal policies and practices at all levels of community (10). Silverman (20, p. 3) reported that when the Black Plague was killing 500 people a day, officials spent time deciding to dig graves six feet deep to prevent fumes from escaping to infect others, instead of being concerned about caring for the sick.

During the HIV/AIDS epidemic, local and federal governments have repeatedly introduced legislation demanding universal, mandatory testing for HIV despite agreement by scientists and economists that such actions were unnecessary, prohibitive in cost and ineffective in controlling the spread of infection (7). Some ministers, and a few politicians, continue to preach that HIV/AIDS is God's punishment for the immoral behavior of homosexuals. The fact that HIV/AIDS in America was prevalent initially among homosexual men and in-

---

[4]Befekadu (1993) was written in French. I am grateful to Drs. Sharon and Mario Valente who transcribed this work into English.

travenous drug users, along with their sexual partners, kindled negative responses among the public, health care providers, and politicians alike.

Since HIV/AIDS is a sexually transmitted disease, discussions of sexual practices are necessary to clarify disease transmission and prevention, but anxiety and taboos have banned open discussions of intimate sexual practices, and impeded effective prevention programs [17]. Unlike many illnesses, sexually transmitted diseases are often perceived as shameful and to be kept private.

Traditionally, nurses, physicians, and other health care workers have tacitly accepted the occupational risk of exposure to serious and fatal illnesses, but antibiotic therapy and other technical advances that have reduced risk of contagion or improved disease management have contributed to a complacency among a whole generation of health care providers. As a result, current health care workers initially acted on their fears more than their compassion, and refused care for those with HIV/AIDS [18]. Although such refusals have grown rare, Marie's experience illustrates a continuing problem. In the early 1990s Marie needed minor surgery to remove a cyst, and was referred to a plastic surgeon in her community. He had completed discussing the treatment and was waiting for confirmation of available scheduling when she asked him if any additional preparations would be needed because of her HIV/AIDS. He had not realized she was HIV positive, and now told her to find another physician. He would not treat anyone who had HIV/AIDS.

The absence of a unified AIDS health plan to guide policy formation and resource development in the USA has resulted in ineffective prevention, unevenly distributed clinical resources, and inconsistent research programs. Other negative reactions include: underfunding research and clinical programs; testing individuals without their consent; evicting people from their homes; restricting immigration of HIV-infected individuals; refusing and canceling health care insurance; excluding people of color, women, and children from scientific studies; and restricting HIV-infected prisoners' access to treatment.

Society's negative reactions enhance potential for individual suffering by increasing the stigma associated with the illness, increasing the burden on the HIV/AIDS individual and family, and limiting the scope of resources a community allocates for the illness [7]. Powell-Cope and Brown [15] found that family caregivers of people with HIV/AIDS also shared the stigma, and experienced intense suffering in the form of rejection, loss of friends, and harassment. Stigma may contribute to strained interpersonal relationships among the patient and supportive others, including family as well as colleagues (10). For example, Hillary's experience reflects how stigma increased her suffering when she was diagnosed with HIV/AIDS. Hillary was visiting her family in the Orient when she learned, to her absolute astonishment, that she was HIV positive. She was in a state of shock for a week, and said nothing to anyone, for she was ashamed of having HIV/AIDS. For Hillary, the diagnosis of HIV/AIDS meant stigma, shame, and death. She said,

> The emotional impact, the trauma, emotional trauma was terrible. It's the worst thing that could happen to anyone. So I finally told my parents about it and of course they were very, very shocked. And I felt so sorry for them because they had so much financial difficulty with their business, and so they already had a lot of problems of their own. Then on top of this I let them know about my problem, and it just about tore them to pieces. So they told me not to eat on the same table, or if I do eat on the same table, not to share. See, back home we all dish out from the same dish. So they told me to have my own bowls and dishes and not to share the eating utensils with them. They don't even allow me to wash my clothes in the sink. And I have to use my own bathroom. I cannot use their bathroom. Things like that. And the worst part is my husband, you know. He, he just totally isolates me.

Stigma also has the potential to intensify negative self-perceptions, which in turn can increase emotional distress, such as depression (10). Because stigma reduces development of clinical and social resources, patients with HIV/AIDS have less access to diagnostic and treatment facilities. Reduced access to care leads to faster disease progression and a shortened lifespan, and both of these are related to suffering.

HIV/AIDS as a Chronic Illness

Once an individual is exposed to HIV, the virus requires a long incubation: six weeks to six months before seroconversion to HIV positive status. Many individuals then have another eight to ten years when they feel relatively well. If HIV/AIDS progresses according to the most common pattern, individuals begin encountering serious opportunistic illnesses only after ten or more years of being infected. In some people the disease HIV/AIDS progresses more rapidly than the norm, while for others, it progresses more slowly.

Being diagnosed with an illness or health problem often triggers patients to change their lifestyle toward healthier behaviors, such as improved diet, stress management, and enhanced physical fitness (24). These lifestyle changes are difficult to maintain over time, as is required for chronic health problems. Sometimes the suffering is prompted by a nagging fear over time, triggered by helplessness and a need to cope with daily problems. Chad spoke of this:

> It was something devastating. In '85 and then into the spring of '86 that was a real terrible time because I felt so helpless. There was absolutely nothing. I knew that I was living with this virus. I knew that I was not going to die next month because of this, but I knew that there was something eating at my insides that I should be consciously [dealing with], and I didn't feel like I has having any assistance.

People grow discouraged with their inability to maintain self-care changes over time. Fred began smoking again after being told he had CMV retinitis and was unable to stop smoking although he tried several times. Tangible, personal, and interpersonal resources (such as energy, health care insurance, social support) that face continued demands over time may become depleted. Depleted hope and resources kindle an individual's fear of becoming a burden on others. Depleted interpersonal resources add to the individual's fear that help will not be forthcoming when needed and that support from meaningful relationships will diminish.

Unfortunately, chronic illness extends over time. As time passes, some things get taken for granted. As people with HIV/AIDS and health care staff become familiar with the characteristics of disease progression, their responses may be routine, complacent, and even harmful. Jake had been very sick for days with constant headaches, constant fevers, and inability to eat much. Doctors responded by ordering the same tests over and over, but not doing anything to help him feel better. Jake said,

> You doctors have been dealing with this so long that you're shell-shocked and you don't always hear the cry for help. [You just say] "Oh well, that's part of HIV. Everybody with HIV/AIDS has those symptoms," and they tend to be ignored on the treatment level until it gets so bad that it's life-threatening.

HIV/AIDS Is Contagious

HIV/AIDS is not spread through casual contact, as are tuberculosis or the common cold. Despite this, people with HIV/AIDS fear being responsible for infecting another person, and many know that they may have infected others before they discovered their HIV positive status. They feel guilty about those possible infections and remorseful about harming others. Jake knew he was responsible for infecting one other person, and this contributed to his decision to remain celibate. Not trusting condoms, Jake could not face the possibility of infecting someone else. Many people with HIV/AIDS are in continuing coupled-relationships, and they have to seek altered, often less satisfying ways of expressing their intimate feelings.

Even when people know their fears of contracting HIV infection through ordinary daily contact are unrealistic, they may continue to harbor some concern. A mother of an adolescent with HIV/AIDS was planning to bring her son home to care for him. She was worried about caring for him because she feared becoming infected. She was ashamed of these fears and voiced concern that she was not a good mother because these fears continued despite medical assurances that she would be safe. Fear of contagion introduces strains in interpersonal relationships, and may contribute to the individual's negative self-concept as a contaminated person. Interpersonal strain and negative self-concept enhance the individual's potential for suffering.

HIV/AIDS Is Incurable

Having no existing cure for HIV/AIDS intensifies the role of uncertainty in a person's living with this chronic illness. HIV/AIDS is among many illnesses without cure, such as diabetes, multiple sclerosis, or alzheimer's disease. While uncertainty can give a person hope for a cure in the future, uncertainty also may impose added burdens on the individual and family. Uncertainty permeates many aspects of living with the illness and its treatment. Chad's experience underscores the combination of uncertainty, daily living and suffering: "Well, the first that I can remember that's definitely HIV related [in the very early 80s] was the skin rash which came so abruptly, was so excruciating, and was undiagnosable." Chad still does not know the cause of his incapacitating skin rash that has never recurred.

Patients have easy access to experimental medications and procedures in clinical trials. Deciding to participate in any clinical trial means making decisions from minimal scientific data. Jake decided to participate in one clinical trial of a growth hormone, and within two weeks the KS that he had struggled to contain had spread rampantly. Not only did he have to withdraw from the study, but also he had to cope with increased physical discomfort from the lesions while wondering if the growth hormone had possibly shortened his life.

Daily living with HIV/AIDS places demands on the person's lifestyle because HIV/AIDS has no cure, and, therefore, no end to uncomfortable procedures and treatments. These treatments are difficult to maintain and, as Chad illustrates, their minor discomforts and forced awareness can be intrusive:

> The daily suffering is the retching with the pills. I mean like last night I took some of my MAI [Mycobacterium avium-intracellulare, or Mycobacterium Avium Complex] meds and one got caught somewhere in my throat and I wasn't really aware of it. I drank the glass of water and all of a sudden I belched and it was this incredible awful toxic mess. I couldn't get rid of that for about an hour and a half regardless of what I gargled with or swallowed. Every day there is taking one or a combination of some of the medications. I think what we are talking about is the awareness of all these. I'm not putting these in and closing my mouth without giving any thought.

Some medications are taken with food; some medications require the person to avoid food for two hours. Planning to have dinner with friends may require that a person reschedule their medication regime for the day. The demands of daily living may impose conditions that, by themselves, are associated with suffering. When the demands occur in the context of an incurable illness, many people extend their perspective automatically to include personal mortality.

HIV/AIDS and Personal Mortality

Being human means that we are mortal—i.e., not only will each of us die, but also we have knowledge that we will die, even though we usually keep this knowledge abstract and distant. Upon learning they have HIV/AIDS, many people respond as Hillary did: they regard the diagnosis as a death sentence. HIV/AIDS brings into awareness our mortality, and this awareness is never very far away for those with HIV/AIDS. Awareness of personal mortality is a key ingredient of suffering. Having been infected before any test could detect HIV, Chad has had many crises with himself and his friends that thrust him toward facing death, and he asked, "How many times have I faced that [death]?" He agreed that each time that he faced some aspect of death, he suffered. Often he also learned something; however, Chad did not believe that he yet fully understood or accepted death. In contrast, Doug talked about Harry who realized the reality of death before he died:

> I visited him [Harry] at the hospital and the night before he had been visited by some premonition of maybe the angel of death and he was terrified. He said that he was very scared. Up until this point he had asked me not to let anybody come to visit him without me there. But now he said, "I've made a terrible, terrible mistake. I've made a mockery of this whole process and what's going on. What's really going on is I'm dying and I'm never going to see these people again unless I see them now."

People with HIV/AIDS fear the suffering that dying will bring and wonder how well they will bear the suffering. Almost all have spoken of how painful it is to watch people they love struggle with pain and dying. For example, Miguel wished that he not get sick and die before his mother because he wanted to spare her the pain of seeing him dead. Still, when his mother became very ill, he told me, "I've been in pain before, but I've never experienced so much pain [as seeing his mother so sick]."

Both Miguel and Doug spoke of their helplessness as they watched loved ones suffer without being able to help. Having no control over the situation is a major ingredient of suffering. Jake spoke of the fact that he could do nothing to let his friend Ken know that Ken could just end his pain and struggling by just letting go. Jake felt helpless because Ken was beyond hearing any message, but Ken's struggling and suffering continued. Jake spoke of his own suffering related to Ken,

> Sometimes I just wake up in the middle of the night just sad, sad. I mean just, not depressed but deeply sad. I mean it's a very painful experience and I don't know how to explain it except it's the ultimate in sad.

Perhaps Jake's sadness over Ken's dying was intensified by the friends as close as family who already were dead: Adrianne, Ken, Michael, Rafael. Jake wondered how much more he could take, and pointed out, "In weeks or months, you know, Jake's not going to be here." In contrast to Jake's willingness to discuss death, others avoid such discussions. For example, Marie's husband is reluctant to talk with her about HIV/AIDS, wills, durable power of attorney, etc. The most he will say is that he can't face the thought of losing her.

A diagnosis of HIV/AIDS brings most people face-to-face with awareness of death. Suffering may emerge from watching others struggle as they either face or avoid death. Reminders of death's toll can be as simple as looking at the growing number of crossed out names in one's address book. When a friend dies, their loved ones and friends suffer from their losses and form re-adjustments in their roles and relationships. Suffering also involves a heightened vulnerability and awareness of one's own mortality, and sometimes a reluctant acknowledgment that one's current hold on life is fragile.

Relief of Suffering

The polemic about suffering is whether suffering is regarded as a distress to be avoided or relieved, or whether suffering is essential to personal growth and development. Rawlinson (16, p. 50) asks, "Ought some sufferings be encouraged, even required, while others are relieved?" Current ethics of health care tend to support the obligation to relieve patient suffering when health care providers have the means to do so (18). Steeves and Kahn (22) linked experiences of suffering with meaning and pointed out that nurses should establish conditions necessary for their patients to experience meaning as a strategy for relieving suffering. Frankl (8) asserted that making sense out of a situation that caused suffering—i.e., finding meaning in the situation—ended the suffering. Without contradicting the possible benefits of suffering, Cassell (3) accuses physicians of neglecting their obligation to relieve suffering because their medical care has been so influenced by Cartesian dualism that splits mind and body. Morse, Bottorff, Anderson, O'Brien, and Solberg (13) argue that nurses must be engaged with their patients to relieve suffering, and they present a model for therapeutic communication strategies. Guidelines do not exist to help nurses, physicians, and other health care providers differentiate purposive and detrimental suffering experiences. This section is organized around a discussion of barriers to relief, providing one's own relief, and receiving relief from others.

Barriers to Relieving Suffering

Most people found barriers to relieving suffering when caring was needed and expected, but not provided. Typically, situations involved disappointment from health care resources, not from family. For example, Jake spoke of the time (p. 20) that he had been so sick for two weeks, and the doctors repeated the same tests,

> They act like they're too busy or that they've got something else on their mind and they're going through the motions of "well, let's order up these tests," and it was always the same test. I was getting frustrated, confused, and very discouraged. For the first time since HIV became a factor in my life, I truly began to believe that these doctors were really going to kill me with their lack of care.

The lack of a sympathetic response from his doctors reinforced Jake's perspective that the staff did not focus on him as a person (13). A different barrier occurred when Hillary became ill while visiting her parents in the Orient. At the hospital, she learned her symptoms were caused by HIV/AIDS. She needed information about HIV/AIDS, available treatment, and her own condition. No information was available; the doctors and nurses knew almost nothing about HIV/AIDS, and Hillary told of not trusting the laboratory test results:

> So of course I cannot trust the T-cell result because they were just starting to do T-cells. So my T-cell turned out to be just fifty-four or something. It was so low. And I could not get hold of AZT. All the private hospitals refused to treat HIV patients. So finally I decided to just rush back here [America].

Both Jake and Hillary described encountering health care staff who increased their confusion, prevented their making sense out of the situation, and also failed to validate their distress.

Sometimes health care staff are so familiar with how a situation will unfold that they don't stop to think about helping patients and families anticipate and plan. Doug spoke of being focused on losing Harry and making him more comfortable during the hospitalization. One of Harry's friends who was a nurse spoke to the hospital staff and discovered that they had stopped all medical interventions and were only providing palliative care. She explained to Doug that the hospital would probably discharge Harry soon to hospice care, and the family needed to investigate resources and make plans. Withholding of information about changes in treatment and the implications for discharge planning made Doug and the family feel as though Harry didn't matter to the staff. They felt overwhelmed.

Another typical situation where the lack of regard for the individual person enhanced the bereaving family/friends' suffering was the funeral, as illustrated by this reaction, "It was strange because at the funeral, and it always enrages, me, there's all this sort of Christian voodoo. No mention of AIDS. No mention of [being gay]. Completely sanitized." People expected the funeral to honor the person who died and to provide relief of their suffering and closure for their grief. When the funeral service fails to acknowledge important dimensions of the person who died, the resulting anger and confusion may enhance and complicate the mourner's process of honoring the deceased person. When friends and relatives perceive that the person they are grieving was devalued at the funeral, instead of being honored, their own grieving and suffering may intensify.

Providing One's Own Relief of Suffering

Finding something to distract attention away from one's suffering may provide temporary relief from suffering. For example, Marie has chronic pain from myositis. While she has attended pain management clinics and uses many of the techniques that she learned, she finds the best relief when she paints. Keeping the same position over time while painting also increases her pain potential, but relieves her suffering. Painting engages and absorbs her attention completely, and this engagement gives her relief. Marie said, "With my painting I could be sitting there for two hours and think it's only half an hour."

Miguel said that his earlier suffering emerged from not dealing with his feelings, and he worked to develop his skills:

> Now I can stop and talk about my feelings and I can start to breathe. As before I did not have those skills and it was just a constant pain. Now I can be nice. I can stop it and do something about it.

Having developed skills to respond to feelings as they arise has given Miguel control over more situations, and has reduced his vulnerability to suffering.

Since feeling out-of-control in a situation is an important element of some suffering experiences, regaining control or reducing helplessness will help relieve suffering. An example of this occurred when Jake, frustrated over his physicians' unwillingness to treat his KS until it was severe, told his physician, "If the KS starts getting worse and my general health starts to deteriorate, I will stop all medication if you don't treat the KS. If you're not going to treat KS, then why should we be treating anything else?" Not only did he take back the power in the situation, but he also found his stand on what mattered to him as he thought through his decision.

Receiving Help from Others to Relieve Suffering

Often, people speak of kind acts from others that provided them with comfort. Chad described how family and friends comforted him when he was discouraged: they listened to him, consoled him when he was tearful, and offered suggestions when he could not find acceptable options.

When the physician told Fred he had CMV, he observed how upsetting this was to Fred. Instead of rushing off to his next appointment, he stayed with Fred for some time. Eventually Fred pointed out to the physician, "I appreciate you being here and I appreciate your trying to help me, but there's not a damn thing anybody else can do. It's something I've got to work through myself." The physician then told the nurses that he was concerned about how upset Fred was, and asked them check on him often. Fred became tearful each time he related this story, and spoke often of how much the physician's actions meant to him, "It meant to me that he really cared. He would do the best for me that he could."

Marie's muscle pain is more intense when she is lying down, and her muscles are tense and achy. She told of her husband's attentiveness, "But my husband massages my neck all the time when it hurts all night, muscles down in here [points to the affected muscle area]. So they're always hurting and then down my arm." Marie receives comfort from the physical effect of the massage and from her husband's patient attentiveness; her first husband was abusive and impatient with her.

Jake described a situation when the help he received from someone else was indirect, but effective in changing the situation that caused his distress and suffering. That time he had been so sick for days, and his physicians kept testing, not treating, him. Jake learned that his therapist had met with the medical staff,

[She] had talked to him [infection disease doctor], and I could tell the difference. The first time he came in the room before he had talked to her [he wasn't interested]—and then he came back later that day, and I mean he was like a totally different person. He was focused on me. He was listening to everything I said, and also, he had more of an openness about him.

Relief of suffering through receiving help from other people was characterized by the sufferers feeling that others cared for them and were engaged with them in the situation. Caring is central for health care professionals in responding to patient suffering (2), (12), (23), (26). Rawlinson (16, p. 60) does not name the process of assistance as caring, but directs us to a different focus, "The goal and guide of our assistance ought always to be the restoration in the subject of the capacity to value, to take ends as his own and pursue them." Alter (1) would add maintaining hope as a focus of assistance.

Alter (1) argued that the experience of illness offers the individual an opportunity to clarify and understand living, and health professionals can play an important role in helping patients and their families develop new understandings of the meaning of illness and new possibilities of hope. Several authors either linked hopelessness with suffering or hope with finding meaning and relieving suffering, or both (21), (9), (6). Cousins (4) spoke of hope as the healing power of the human spirit because hope functions as a challenge. In her qualitative study of maintaining hope in HIV disease, Hall (9) portrayed the maintenance of hope as pivotal in balancing suffering, and she called for health care to build structures to support patients' efforts. One way that health professionals can relieve suffering is by helping patients find meaning within the experience of being ill, and hope may be an important channel (4), (6). Support of hope by health care providers requires that patients' wishes be considered, and care be delivered in ways that do not compound the suffering of HIV/AIDS (9).

Summary

HIV/AIDS has many features that increase potential for suffering in those touched by this illness. Society's reaction to this illness and to the people stigmatized by it has been negative and judgmental, resulting in individual discrimination and inadequate community responses. Chronicity of the illness depletes personal resources. Awareness of personal mortality is always close. Suffering, the distress felt by the person in response to disharmony within the self, represents a rupture between the situation and those ends that matter. Living with HIV/AIDS is a dance of complex—sometimes contradictory—rhythms, not constant suffering, as illustrated by Chad,

> My life is graced and I am blessed and part of my blessing is having HIV/AIDS, and I know it's a terrible disease. Sometimes I don't even want to live with myself with all of this going on. In fact, I'm very unhappy because it also totally changes my life. My retirement isn't over, but I think I am really cheated.

References

1. Alter, C. L. (1994). Redefining hope in the second decade of AIDS: A psychiatrist's experience. *AIDS Patient Care, 8,* 2–5.
2. Befekadu, E. (1993). La souffrance: Clarification conceptuelle. *Canadian Journal of Nursing Research, 25,* 7–21.
3. Cassell, E. J. (1982). The nature of suffering and the goals of medicine. *The New England Journal of Medicine, 306,* 639–645.
4. Cousins, N. (1989). *Head first: The biology of hope and the healing power of the human spirit.* New York: Penguin Books.
5. Durham, J. D. (1994). The changing HIV/AIDS epidemic: Emerging psychosocial challenges for nurses. In D. F. Pennebaker (Ed.), *Mental health nursing in nursing clinics of North America.* Philadelphia: W. B. Saunders & Co.
6. Farran, C. J., Herth, K. A., & Popovich, J. M. (In Press). *Hope and hopelessness: Critical clinical constructs.* Newbury Park, CA: Sage Publications.
7. Flaskerud, J. H. (1992). Psychosocial aspects. In J. H. Flaskerud & P. J. Ungvarski (Eds.), *HIV/AIDS A guide to nursing care* (pp. 239–274). Philadelphia: W. B. Saunders.
8. Frankl, V. (1972). *Man's search for meaning.* New York: Pocket Books.
9. Hall, B. A. (1994). Ways of maintaining hope in HIV disease. *Research in Nursing & Health, 17,* 283–293.
10. Herek, G. M., & Glunt, E. K. (1988). An epidemic of stigma. *American Psychologist, 43,* 886–891.
11. Kahn, D. L., & Steeves, R. H. (1986). The experience of suffering: A concept clarification and theoretical definition. *Journal of Advanced Nursing, 11,* 623–631.
12. Lindholm, L., & Erikson, K. (1993). To understand and alleviate suffering in a caring community. *Journal of Advanced Nursing, 18,* 1354–1361.
13. Morse, J. M., Bottorff, J., Anderson, G., O'Brien, B., & Solberg, S. (1992). Beyond empathy: Expanding expressions of caring. *Journal of Advanced Nursing, 17,* 809–821.
14. O'Brien, M. E. (1992). *Living with HIV. Experiment in courage.* New York: Auburn House.
15. Powell-Cope, G. M., & Brown, M. A. (1992)., Going public as an AIDS family caregiver. *Social Science and Medicine, 5,* 571–580.

16. Rawlinson, M. C. (1986). The sense of suffering. *Journal of Medicine and Philosophy, 11,* 39–62.
17. Saunders, J. M., & Underwood, P. J. (1991). HIV infection: Helping adolescents choose safer behaviors. *Journal of Child and Adolescent Psychiatric and Mental Health Nursing, 4,* 132–136.
18. Saunders, J. M. (In press). Ethical issues related to the care of persons with HIV. In J. H. Flaskerud & P. J. Ungvarski (Eds.), *HIV/AIDS: A guide to nursing care,* Third Edition. Philadelphia: W. B. Saunders.
19. Saunders, J. M. (1991). Nursing management of persons with disease about which little is known: Prototype—AIDS. In S. B. Baird, R. McCorkle, & M. Grant (Eds.), *Cancer nursing: A comprehensive textbook* (pp. 708–716). Philadelphia: W. B. Saunders.
20. Silverman, M. F. (1990). The social and political impact of the AIDS epidemic. *AIDS Patient Care,* 3–7.
21. Spross, J. A. (1993). Pain, suffering, and spiritual well-being: Assessment and interventions. *Quality of life. A Nursing Challenge, 2,* 71–79.
22. Steeves, R. H., & Kahn, D. L. (1987). Experience of meaning in suffering. *Image: Journal of Nursing Scholarship, 19,* 114–116.
23. Travelbee, J. (1971). *Interpersonal Aspects of Nursing.* Philadelphia: F. A. Davis.
24. Valente, S. M., Saunders, J. M., & Uman, G. (1993). Self-care, psychological distress, and HIV disease. *Journal of the Association of Nurses and AIDS Care, 6,* 15–25.
25. Watson, J. (1979). *Nursing: The philosophy and science of caring.* Boulder, CO: Colorado Associated University Press.
26. Watson, J. (1985). *Nursing: Human science and human care: A theory of nursing.* Norwalk, CT: Appleton-Century-Crofts.
27. *Webster's Third New International Dictionary of the English Languaged,* Unabridged. (1986). Springfield, Mass.: Merriam-Webster, Inc. (p. 2284).

Chapter 5

Suffering and Survivorship

Mel Haberman, PhD, RN   *Director of Research,*

Oncology Nursing Society

Introduction

> Critical illness leaves no aspect of life untouched. . . . [The patient]
> will suffer and have losses, but suffering and loss are not incom-
> patible with life. For all you lose, you have an opportunity to gain:
> closer relationships, more poignant appreciations, clarified values.
> You are entitled to mourn what you can no longer be, but do not
> let this mourning obscure your sense of what you can become.
> You are embarking on a dangerous opportunity. Do not curse your
> fate; count your possibilities (1, p. 7).

Cancer screening and early detection activities and new advances
in therapy have steadily increased the number of cancer survivors. In
1994, over 8 million Americans were living with a history of cancer
and over 5 million were diagnosed 5 or more years ago (2). The
American Cancer Society (2) estimates that 40 percent of all persons
diagnosed with cancer in 1994 will be alive 5 years after diagnosis.
When adjusted for normal life expectancy and factors such as dying of
heart disease, accidents, and diseases of old age, the relative 5-year
survival rate for all cancers is 53 percent. Cancers with a steadily
improving relative 5-year survival rate are listed in Table 5–1.

Despite the encouraging news that the 5-year survival rate for
many types of cancer is improving, traditional indicators of cancer
survival, such as relapse rates and length of disease-free survival, tell
us little about the nature or quality of survival after cancer therapy (3).
Gottheil and colleagues (4) support the current viewpoint that the mere
preservation of life is no longer a satisfactory sole criterion of the
outcome of treatment, however, they cautioned, "variables such as
hope, the will to live, and the quality of life have not been readily
amenable to objective investigation" (p. 632). Recent advances in the
measurement of quality of life have led to a growing consensus among
health care providers, cancer advocates, and cancer survivors. Namely,
any evaluation of the effectiveness of therapy must now include such
factors as quality of life and the psychosocial aspects of survivorship.
Consequently, an expanded definition of cancer survivorship is rapidly

The author wishes to acknowledge Linda Eaton, MN, RN, OCN, and Kelli Wisdom for
their assistance in the preparation of the manuscript. Mel Haberman is an employee of
the Oncology Nursing Society. The Oncology Nursing Society assumes no responsibility
for the content of this publication.

TABLE 5–1   Cancers with Increasing 5-Year Relative Survival Rate

Type of Cancer	Percent White	Percent Black
All sites	55	39
Testicular cancer	93	84
Thyroid gland	92	92
Melanoma of skin	84	72
Breast cancer	81	64
Urinary/bladder cancer	80	61
Hodgkin's disease	79	74
Prostate cancer	79	64
Colon cancer	60	49
Rectal cancer	58	45
Ovarian cancer	40	40
Leukemia	39	30

Source: American Cancer Society, *Cancer Facts & Figures* (2)

emerging that recognizes the salience of quality of life and not just quantity of life.

With a whole new set of factors for gauging the quality of survival after cancer therapy, newly diagnosed persons and their families routinely transform their mathematical probability for survival into personal terms. Quality of life issues act to humanize the statistical odds so the survival projection will more appropriately fit the individual's unique life situation (5). In addition to asking, "What are my chances of being cured?," it is now commonplace for newly diagnosed persons to weigh the advantages and disadvantages of various therapies by asking, "How will the different treatments affect my ability to work, play with my children, enjoy my hobbies, and spend quality time with my family and friends?"

The purpose of this chapter is to review some of the current definitions of cancer survivorship and to identify some of the life, disease, and treatment-related issues that influence the suffering experienced by persons with cancer. Emphasis is placed on the biopsychosocial issues that are prevalent during the early diagnostic period and the extended (remission) or permanent (cure) stages of survival. Definitions of survivorship are now provided to identify some of the common meanings given to the term, *cancer survivorship*.

Definitions of Survivorship

> It was desperate days of nausea and depression. It was elation at
> the birth of a daughter in the midst of treatment. It was the anxiety
> of waiting for my monthly chest film to be taken and lying awake
> nights feeling for lymph nodes. It was the joy of eating Chinese
> food for the first time after battling radiation burns of the esopha-
> gus for four months. These reflections . . . are a jumble of memories
> of a purgatory that was touched by sickness in all its aspects but
> was neither death nor cure. It was survival (6, p. 271).

One challenge in understanding the issues of cancer survivorship
is agreeing on a definition. Survivorship has been described in various
ways including an ill-defined condition (6); a process of biopsychosocial
transition that extends continuously through time (7); and an ongoing,
continuum of life that extends through and beyond the illness experience (8). Survivorship has traditionally been linked to some predetermined time period, such as living to the 2- or 5-year milepost after the
initial diagnosis or the end of therapy. Leigh and colleagues (8) note
that definitions of survival have historically been limited to individuals
deemed "cured" of their primary disease, with cure being defined as
having "no evidence of disease with a minimal or nonexistent chance
for recurrence" (8, p. 485). The American Cancer Society regards a
person as statistically "cured" when there is a total lack of any evidence
of disease and the individual has the same life expectancy as someone
who never had cancer (2). To overcome the inherent limitation of
previous definitions of survivorship that are time-bound and emphasize
cure as the sole criterion of successful therapy, the National Coalition
for Cancer Survivorship (NCCS) offers a broader definition of cancer
survivorship: "From the time of its discovery and for the balance of
life, an individual diagnosed with cancer is a survivor" (9, p. 2).

The NCCS definition expands the notion of survivorship by shift-
ing the emphasis from the cure of cancer to therapeutic goals that place
a value on caring behaviors and outcomes of symptom control, palliation, and comfort. This broader definition of survivorship more accu-
rately reflects the natural history of cancer and treatment. Cancer is
not a single disease entity but varies by onset, tumor staging, dissemination, prognosis and treatability (10). It often has no clear onset or
easily predicted course and the outcome of therapy may be uncertain.
Many cancers, such as skin or early detected prostate cancer are often
cured following surgical intervention and the individual may be con-

sidered cured long before the 5-year survival milepost (8). Other cancers, such as lung, multiple myeloma and liver cancer, have a low probability of cure.

Definitions of survivorship must also account for the differential goals and trajectories of various cancer therapies such as surgery, radiation, chemotherapy, biological therapy, and bone marrow transplantation. Used singularly or in combination, cancer therapies often generate a host of side-effects that place survivors at risk to varying degrees of biopsychosocial morbidity and, in some cases, premature death from the iatrogenic effects of therapy. Consequently, unlike many illnesses where people feel better after diagnosis and treatment, the reverse is often true with cancer (7).

Many cancer survivors dread the sequelae of cancer therapy, even if successful. Recovery is not a linear process; one does not generally get better and better each day, but improvement comes in spurts and with frequent setbacks (11). Fearing the debilitating side effects of therapy and/or the potential for treatment failure, many survivors turn to the use of alternative or nontraditional forms of cancer therapy (12), (13). Other persons who are initially diagnosed as "incurable" and given little, if any, hope for cure, may decline all forms of therapy or opt to undergo palliative care. In the presence of progressive disease or in the terminal stages of illness, therapy may be targeted at controlling the spread of cancer, maximizing physical comfort, and buying time to put one's affairs in order and say one's good-byes. Individuals who will not achieve a cure, in a strict medical sense, are nonetheless survivors of a chronic illness condition (8). Lastly, an exceptional group of survivors exists, namely, individuals thought to be terminal who, against all medical expectations, experience a full recovery, a miracle cure, or spontaneous remission (8), (14).

The different trajectories of cancer survivorship and the increasing longevity of life after cancer diagnosis have resulted in cancer being redefined as a chronic, life-threatening illness rather than a terminal disease (7), (8). In a study of individuals who had survived from 1 to 33 years after therapy, Shanfield (15) found that cancer survivorship is, in fact, a permanent life experience. Many years or decades after the completion of therapy, the survivors easily recalled the initial despair associated with the acute phase of illness, expressed continuing concerns for their mortality, and reported an enduring sense of vulnerability to recurrence. In another study of 10 individuals who were between 3 and 15 years postdiagnosis, Eakes (16) documented periodic episodes of sadness and feelings of grief both in survivors with active disease and in those who were disease-free, indicating the permanent nature of chronic sorrow in cancer survivors. Eakes concluded that chronic sorrow should be viewed as a normal response to the chronicity of cancer survivorship. Since the sadness was cyclic in nature, the persons were able to experience periods of satisfaction and happiness and were not considered debilitated by their chronic sorrow. Grief-related feelings were most often triggered by scheduled visits for routine follow-up examinations, the presence of physical discomfort, reminders of the losses associated with the diagnosis, and the uncertainty of living with cancer. Clearly, any definition of survivorship must reflect the chronicity and natural history of cancer, the wide variety of potential treatment outcomes, and the types of biopsychosocial morbidity experienced by survivors. Based on the aforementioned factors that shape a broader conceptualization of cancer survivorship, the phases of survivorship are now described.

Phases of Survival

There is widespread agreement in the literature that survivorship is an evolutionary or developmental process rather than a discrete event that occurs at some predetermined time, such as living 5 years beyond diagnosis [6], [7], [8], [17], [18], [19], [20]. Parkes [21] used the term "psychosocial transitions" to conceptualize chronic illnesses, like cancer, as dynamic and ongoing life experiences. A full understanding of the natural history of cancer, then, can only be obtained by delineating the nature of these transitions or passages and the challenges and hardships that characterize each phase of survivorship [7]. Stage-theories or models of cancer survivorship can assist clinicians in their efforts to give anticipatory guidance to patients and families [5] and to develop research agendas that focus on identifying the specific needs of persons with cancer at various points in the illness trajectory [6].

Several conceptual models have been proposed to describe the continuum of cancer survivorship. Mages and Mendelsohn [7] identified several phases of survivorship: discovery and diagnosis of the cancer; primary treatment; remission with a return to normal activity; and, in some cases, recurrence and dissemination; and terminal illness. Similarly, Fiore [19] delineated six phases of cancer therapy based on his own experience with cancer and surgical intervention. The phases include the initial time of diagnosis, preoperative care, postoperative recovery and adjustment to the loss of physical function or a body part, postoperative therapy, the termination of active therapy or the rehabilitation phase, and the post five-year survival period.

In a well-known model of survivorship, Mullan (6) identified three longitudinal phases of survivorship—acute, extended, permanent—which he called "seasons of survival." The acute season begins at the time of diagnosis. This period is dominated by the medical aspects of obtaining diagnostic confirmation and undertaking primary or adjuvant therapy. Fear, anxiety, and pain are common elements of this stage as well as a personal confrontation with one's own mortality. Mullan (6) commented, "Simply coping with the effects of the therapies occupies all the adaptive energies of most patients" during the initial phase of survivorship (p. 271).

The extended stage of survival follows the initial phase. This phase begins when the first course of therapy is completed or when the individual goes into remission. The hallmarks of the extended phase are "watchful waiting," periodic follow-up examinations, consolidation or maintenance therapy, diminished physical endurance, fatigue, and re-entry at home and work. Psychologically, this phase is dominated by the fear or recurrence, altered body image and, perhaps, a different vocational or school role. Depression, devastation, social isolation, and anxiety are common.

Mullan noted that the last, permanent stage of survivorship is roughly equated with achieving a cure. However, Mullan (6) indicated that "there is no moment of cure but rather an evolution from the phase of extended survival into a period when the . . . disease or the likelihood of its return is sufficiently small that the cancer can now be considered permanently arrested" (p. 272). Problems with employment; health and life insurance; reproductive health for young people; and potential secondary effects of cancer characterize this phase of survivorship.

The various stage models of cancer survivorship tend to complement one another by using different terms to describe essentially the same or similar aspects of survival. Conceptualizing cancer survivorship as a continuum of overlapping stages provides a developmental framework for identifying the biopsychosocial issues that emerge over the course of a lifetime (8).

Biopsychosocial Issues

Mages and Mendelsohn (7) organized the psychosocial effects of cancer around three general propositions: (a) cancer survivorship is an ongoing life experience that unfolds over a considerable period of time, (b) the personal changes produced by cancer must be understood within the context of the individual's life stage and history, and (c) the psychosocial issues that emerge at any given time are the result of the person's need to adapt to the biophysical realities of the illness. Weisman and Worden (10) echo the sentiment that the most salient factor that determines how people adjust to living with cancer is the concrete nature of the disease.

Holland (18) delineates several clinical pathways that influence the psychosocial aspects of cancer survivorship. The clinical pathways may include (a) long-term survival and cure, (b) some period of disease-free survival followed by recurrence, (c) primary treatment failure and disease progression, and (d) situations where no curative treatment is possible so therapy focuses on control and palliation.

Holland (18) identified the psychosocial issues that occur during the clinical course of cancer, beginning with the diagnostic work-up phase of survivorship. The diagnosis and workup for cancer actually begin when the person finds a suspicious sign of cancer and makes the decision to seek diagnostic confirmation. In addition to confronting the possibility of having cancer, the person may not want to prematurely alarm their family, preferring to carry the burden of the suspected diagnosis and fear alone. Moreover, people will recall prior family experiences with cancer, especially earlier times when cancer therapy or comfort measures were limited or accompanied with gruesome pain and suffering. Providing psychosocial support to the person and their family is essential during this period as well as ensuring that accurate information is provided in a timely fashion. Individual reactions to the diagnosis may range from fear, shock and disbelief, concerns about disfigurement, and anger to a sense of relief that an explanation for one's symptoms has finally been found and therapy can begin (5). Weisman and Worden (10) coined the term "existential plight" to refer to the distress of this period. Existential plight is characterized by optimism that therapy will result in cure; some transient functional impairment; and the use of denial, cognitive, and behavioral strategies to manage emotional distress.

The next phase of the clinical course of cancer begins with the initiation of primary treatment, usually multimodal therapy consisting of surgery, radiation, chemotherapy or immunotherapy (18). The individual must give informed consent, manage the side-effects of therapy, maintain high morale, and cooperate with health providers so the entire course of treatment can be given (18). Waiting for the initiation of treatment can be highly anxious for patients and their families (5), (18). Individuals are at risk of psychological exhaustion from a prolonged course of therapy and/or severe illness. In the event of treatment failure and progressive disease, central concerns during the terminal phase of care include the psychological and ethical issues that surround the decision to write a "do not resuscitate" order; other end-of-life issues that require shared decision-making by the team of care providers, patient and family members; and providing comfort measures to control pain and minimize protracted suffering (18).

Beliefs in Personal Control

Another psychosocial aspect of cancer survivorship is the threat cancer imposes on all realms of life including people's beliefs in an orderly and controllable world (5). Upon receiving the diagnosis of cancer, there is a universal response that life itself is threatened and that life is now precarious and unpredictable (22), (23). Regaining a belief in a comprehensible world often begins with the confirmation of a definitive diagnosis and the initiation of therapy. Fiore (22) remarked: "When the diagnosis of cancer is rendered, the sense of chaos, fear, and loss of control can be so great that patients and their families will often attribute to the disease special meaning in an attempt to support their belief in an orderly world" (p. 34). Persons with cancer will often seek to regain their belief in a controllable world by searching for some logical explanation for the cause of the disease (5), (24), (25), (26). For instance, persons with leukemia undergoing bone marrow transplantation identified several causes for the disease including exposure to toxic chemicals or microwave radiation, heredity and genetic predisposition, God's will, and a stressful lifestyle (27).

Finding a causal explanation for why cancer occurred is often the first step in preventing a feared recurrence (25). Moreover, coping with the impact of cancer may be facilitated by the person's ability to distinguish various dimensions of control, such as control over life in general and control related specifically to one's health state (28). For example, in a study by Lewis and colleagues (29), persons in the terminal stage of cancer identified four general ways for expressing control during the end-stage of life: monitoring their daily progress and health status, surrendering the struggle for control and passively waiting for death, the use of cognitive strategies such as explaining and re-interpreting to refocus control, and turning over control to family members and health providers. In another study, women with breast cancer perceived themselves as having control over the disease when they used techniques for psychological control such as meditation, imagery, and positive thinking (23).

Fear of Recurrence and Recurrent Disease

The fear of disease recurrence is another psychosocial issue that is a ubiquitous concern of cancer survivors (6), (7), (11), (20), (24), (25), (31), (32), (33). Recurrence is often regarded as more distressing than initial diagnosis since it signifies a loss of hope, the person's failure, or the failure of health providers to halt the downward course of the disease (7), (31), (32), (33). The widely held assumptions that recurrence is more devastating than the initial diagnosis of cancer and that persons with recurrent disease experience more problems compared to those without recurrence may not hold true for all persons with recurrent disease (17). Weisman and Worden (34), in a study that compared 102 persons with recurrent cancer with 102 newly diagnosed persons with the same types of cancer, reported that 30% of the individuals with recurrent disease found the experience less stressful than their original diagnosis. Several factors helped the individuals to manage the distress of recurrence, such as being more familiar with the cancer care system the second time around, a better understanding of therapy and the side-effects of treatment, and having more resources for support.

Schmale (32) observed that recurrent disease opens old psychological wounds and makes the person's "worst fears of what could possibly happen," now become a stark reality. Persons with recurrent disease often feel powerless and helpless as they worry about the impact of the cancer on their career, intimate relationships and bodily functions, and as they reconfront their own mortality and the unpredictability of their future (7). The fear of relapse may present in many forms, ranging from a diffuse uneasiness at the appearance of a new symptom to full-blown panic attacks (8). Discovering a new lump, a sore throat, a suspicious looking patch of skin—anything which cannot be readily explained or regarded as normal—can become the source of fear and serious concern (11). Moreover, efforts to assess or self-monitor suspicious symptoms may actually heighten fears of recurrence when symptoms are ambiguous and uninterpretable (25).

The fear of recurrence often exacerbates just prior to regularly scheduled follow-up visits or at hearing the news that a friend or loved one has been diagnosed with cancer, relapsed, or died of the disease. Mullan (35) indicated that the fear of recurrence should be expected by all persons with cancer as a normal aspect of the recovery process. Openly acknowledging that recurrence will probably happen "will reduce anxiety, minimize loneliness, and make the path to survivorship an easier one" (35, p. 89). Individuals who report an awareness of being at risk to recurrence are less likely to suffer from symptoms of stress when recurrence actually occurs than persons who are completely surprised by the recurrence (31), (32), (33). Cella and colleagues (33) reported that people who believed they were cured and no longer vulnerable to recurrence were prone to stress symptoms of depression, anxiety, intrusive dreams, heightened stress arousal, and social withdrawal, upon learning of the recurrence. Similarly, Mahon (31) indicated that remission is an ambiguous situation that becomes problematic when the person begins to worry that time is marked and running short, and that sooner or later the remission will end.

The person with recurrent disease must cope with re-entering the cancer care system. Moreover, recurrence brings new physical symptoms, disabling therapy, pain, progressive debility, and, quite possibly, death (7). Frequently, the experience of going through the initial course of therapy will discourage people to the point that they would rather let the recurrent disease run its course than endure a new round of treatment (32). Such individuals, particularly those who previously experienced many regimen-related toxicities, now know exactly what to expect from retreatment. Treatment is no longer an unknown, but a dreaded reality. The person may question, "Is it worth going through therapy again, being that sick again?" They may state, "I now know what to expect and I'm not sure I can go through it again." It's important for nurses to identify how people with recurrent disease perceived their initial therapy and to be able to listen to the individual's fears about their inability to endure another cycle of retreatment. One educational resource that is available free of charge is the publication entitled, "When Cancer Recurs: Meeting the Challenge Again," published by The United States Department of Health and Human Services, National Institute of Health (36).

Many people initially say they will never undergo cancer therapy again only to change their minds and opt for retreatment. Often times, older persons with recurrent cancer believe the initial therapy gave them the added time they wanted to enjoy life, therefore, they are reluctant to undertake further treatment, especially if they anticipate further discomfort and physical decline (32). Care providers must balance the importance of giving accurate information with the necessity to sustain hope when people with recurrent disease are confronted with the inevitability of a poor prognosis (31), (32), (33). In noting that "all survivors go through extended periods in which they cannot be sure that they are disease-free," Mullan (35) concluded that there is no substitute for "good, clean diagnostic and prognostic information" (p. 89).

Recurrence is often a time of confusion characterized by a re-activated search for meaning. In a study of 72 individuals who were diagnosed with recurrent disease within 21 months prior to the study, Johnston-Taylor (24) documented that high symptom distress and increased social dependency are associated with an unclear sense of meaning. Moreover, a lack of clear meaning was related to poor psychosocial adjustment. The longer the people lived with recurrent disease, the more unclear their sense of meaning or purpose in life became. However, without knowing the individuals' sense of meaning prior to diagnosis, it's not known if the recurrent cancer either strained or strengthened the survivors' sense of meaning (24).

Future Concerns, Re-Entry Issues, and Re-Establishing a New Normalcy

The permanent impact and lasting importance of cancer is nowhere more evident than survivors' concerns about the future. From the moment of diagnosis, life becomes provisional for the cancer survivor. A lingering sense of uncertainty may pervade every aspect of life, accompanied by fears of a shortened life span and unpredictable future. Survivors are often unable to engage in future-oriented activity as they end therapy and make the transition of moving forward with their lives (11). Maher (11) stated, "The more a patient has learned to 'live for today' during the treatment period, the more he or she is likely to be adrift when faced with the prospect of a tomorrow" (p. 911). The future may be foreshortened to the narrow time span between bouts of acute nausea, to the interval between treatment cycles, or to the time between active episodes of disease (11).

Many long-term survivors maintain a cautious skepticism about their future health and express concerns about their family's future. Survivors may worry about the long-term effects of receiving chemotherapy and radiation, such as the possibility of manifesting a secondary malignancy. They may worry about the family's ability to handle a recurrence or fear they will become a burden to the family in the future. People may wonder if they will live long enough to see their children grow up, about their ability to provide financial security for their loved ones, and whether their children are genetically predisposed to developing cancer (37). Survivors who continue to experience the lingering physical complications of therapy may worry about their body's ability to handle old age, illustrating that cancer survivorship is always embedded within the broader context of life and superimposed on the normal aging process.

Getting on with living and establishing a new normalcy to life are prominent aspects of recovery from cancer (25), (37). Many people are surprised when cancer survivors actually return from what is generally seen as a death sentence (38). Problems of re-entry occur to almost all survivors who undergo a period of remission after a diagnosis of cancer (35). Most of the challenges of re-entry occur within the first five years, making these years a prime time for implementing targeted educational strategies to enhance the nature and quality of re-entry (35). Survivors must learn to reenter the world of the living and compensate for the limitations imposed by the lingering complications of the disease and therapy. Life may take on a new sense of urgency as survivors rebuild and stabilize their lives (25). Rarely, if ever, does life return completely back to normal. Maher (11) recounted the story of one cancer survivor who stated, "Getting well did not mean 'back to normal,' in the old sense, because 'there wasn't any normal to come back to—you were different, other people were different" (p. 909).

The impact of cancer on the ability to return to work and/or school, hiring and job retention discrimination, mistreatment in the workplace, and the actual or potential loss of job productivity are major re-entry issues facing millions of cancer survivors (8), (20), (30), (39), (40). Leigh and colleagues (8) commented that employment discrimination problems can be attributed to three prevalent myths about cancer; namely, that cancer is generally perceived as a death sentence, cancer is a contagious disease even in situations where a cure is achieved, and survivors are perceived as unproductive in the workplace. Employment problems may include dismissal, demotion, failure to hire or promote, a loss of work-related benefits (8), (39), social avoidance, shunning by co-workers, and hostility in the workplace (3), (27), (35), (39). Certain federal and state laws prohibit job discrimination against cancer survivors and disabled persons in general (e.g., the Federal Rehabilitation Act of 1973 and the Americans with Disabilities Act (8)).

Studies have generally reported that 15 to 40 percent of long-term survivors experience physical limitations and lingering side-effects of therapy (3), (30). However, there is little evidence to support the widely held misconceptions that cancer survivors are plagued by psychological or physical hindrances that jeopardize their work performance (30) and that survivors are less productive than other workers (39). Cella (30) notes that problems of work discrimination and job re-entry are probably disease specific and work-site dependent, e.g., following surgical intervention, a lack of physical stamina may affect blue collar workers more than sedentary office workers who underwent the same therapy. In a recent study of individuals who had survived from six to eighteen years after bone marrow transplant, 75 percent of the recipients had returned to full or part-time employment (3). Although 90 percent of the marrow transplant survivors had health insurance (3), life and health insurance discrimination is a common problem facing cancer survivors (8), (30), (39), (40). Survivors may also experience a sense of personal vulnerability due to financial and job insecurity and health or life insurance discrimination (40). Nurses can support the efforts of cancer service organizations and advocacy groups who lobby for cancer survivors and their career, social and economic protection (39), (40).

Serendipitous Benefits of the Cancer Experience

Survivors often report many serendipitous benefits of the cancer experience, such as feeling fortunate to be alive, expressing a greater appreciation for life, and feeling more satisfied with their overall quality of life (3), (8), (15), (25), (41). Quite often, survivors radically change their lifestyle as a reaction to the possibility of a premature death (8), (25). Survivors often reassess their life goals, re-examine their career aspirations, and refocus their priorities (15), (37), (42), (43), (44). No longer taking life for granted, survivors often perceive themselves as more compassionate, grateful, understanding, and patient with others, as the result of the cancer experience. They learn to live life with a shortened time perspective, taking each day as it comes, "living day-by-day."

Social Support Issues

Adaptation to cancer necessitates the re-ordering of social relationships (42), (43), (44), (45), (46). Efforts to re-align social relationships often require the construction of new or expanded social networks, often involving a mixture of formal community agencies and informal survivor support groups (20). However, despite the need to form new relationships and obtain tangible aide and emotional support from others, many cancer survivors experience social isolation, loneliness, and a stigmatized identity (37). Mullan (35) remarks that social "shunning . . . is the scourge of cancer patients" (p. 91). In a study of marrow transplant recipients who had lived from six to eighteen years after transplant, long-term survivors reported that other people became less supportive over time (3). In fact, diminished social support was the single most frequently mentioned and most stressful hardship of long-term survivorship.

    Psychosocial support undoubtedly has a positive influence on the way persons with cancer and their families adjust to the illness (47). Spiegel (47) notes that social integration is associated with reduced mortality from cancer. Support groups are effective in improving the way patients and families cope with such issues as work discrimination, family stress, fears of recurrence, pain managemnent, symptom control, childhood cancer, and the emotional issues that surround terminal care. Clearly, nurses can encourage persons with cancer to join or instigate a support group, if a support group is deemed appropriate for the person or family. Mutual support and cancer advocacy programs such as the American Cancer Society's "I Can Cope" Program, "The Candelighter's Foundation," and "Reach for Recovery" programs are offered in many communities. Several newsletters exist to help survivors and family members including "The Networker," published by the National Coalition for Cancer Survivorship (48) and "The BMT Newsletter," published by Susan Stewart (49). Two excellent references that identify national support programs and community resources for cancer survivors are entitled, *Facing Forward: A Guide for Cancer Survivors* (50) and the book, *Triumph: Getting Back to Normal When You Have Cancer* (51).

Research Issues

Although a great deal of clinical anecdotal information and personal stories of survivorship exist in the scientific and lay literature, little systematic research has been conducted on the psychosocial nature of survivorship. Similarly, even though much is known about the physical late effects of therapy, less is known about the psychosocial sequelae of survivorship (38). As new cancer therapies are developed, understanding their impact on the quality of life of persons with cancer both during and after treatment becomes crucial (52). Mullan (6) stated, "As we move from an earlier time when few cancers were treated successfully to the point when virtually all of them will be cured, we are passing through an uncharted middle ground, which in many aspects remains primitive. The challenge in overcoming cancer is not only to find therapies that will prevent or arrest the disease quickly but also to map the middle ground of survivorship and minimize its medical and social hazards" (p. 273).

Research is also needed on the social implications of cancer. How do persons with cancer and their families or caregivers define social support? What type of support is needed at different points in the disease and treatment trajectory? How can self-help support groups be structured to enhance the coping ability of persons with cancer? Other social implications include the need to better understand our cultural beliefs and societal attitudes towards cancer, e.g., beliefs about cancer contagion, survivors' productivity in the workpkace, and the enduring misconception that cancer is an automatic death sentence.

Additional research on the quality of life of cancer survivors is essential to improving our understanding of the suffering experienced by short and long-term survivors of cancer. More research is needed to demonstrate the efficacy of various self-care behaviors—exercise, diet, biofeedback, relaxation and meditation techniques—and their ability to modulate the stressors of survivorship, reduce uncertainty, and increase a sense of personal control (20). A better understanding of the developmental aspects of cancer is needed. Little is known about the effects of cancer therapy on the normal aging process and the long-term cognitive alterations that occur following chemotherapy and radiation.

Another area of research involves the types of educational and support programs needed to facilitate biopsychosocial adaptation throughout the entire continuum of survivorship. Issues of psychosocial morbidity are especially critical with the recurrence of cancer and/or during progressive disease. A clearer delineation is needed of the nursing interventions that occur when therapy is aimed at cure versus palliation and symptom control. Lastly, research is needed to compare the physical and psychosocial outcomes of cancer therapy with the outcomes of other types of chronic illness, and to compare the long-range adjustment of cancer survivors with people who have never been diagnosed with cancer.

Conclusion

This chapter has briefly surveyed some of the unique issues facing cancer survivors. Cella (30) remarked that the "problems of the cancer survivor are not mere extensions of the problems of the cancer patient in treatment" (p. 66). Survivors face the normal problems of living just like other people with one essential difference. Cancer survivorship poses additional burdens, e.g., managing the physical sequelae of therapy, re-entry into the family and workplace, and the fear of recurrence and progressive disease, to name a few. As the number of cancer survivors steadily increases due to improved screening and early detection programs and new multi-modal therapies, the need to better understand the quality of life of cancer survivors will grow as will the need to develop programs to overcome the unique problems of survivorship.

This chapter began with a quotation by Frank who described the "dangerous opportunities and possibilities" available to cancer survivors. The chapter closes with a similar quotation by Ellen Bushkin, former Chair of the Oncology Nursing Foundation. "Signposts of survival" was the metaphor chosen by Ellen to depict the many twists and turns that guided her journey along the path of survivorship, as she and her family lived life to the fullest, despite the looming presence of cancer. What it means to be a cancer survivor "for the balance of life" is told eloquently:

The journey is exhausting, and still the ultimate sign has not been revealed; you still do not know where the road has taken you. . . . The journey changes your personality, your value structure, your capabilities, and your insights into your life and the lives of others. The journey is a gift of hope, strength, and most of all truth. You and the traveler begin to gain wondrous insight into the value of living and the precious gifts of time, love, and guides. . . . The traveler no longer sees Insurmountable Odds as an inevitable final stop but instead realizes that there are Endless Possibilities for living a life of endurance, hope, and courage. The illness is only a small part of the mission, the message of the journey was that there are many positive signposts along the road to change the way we look at Insurmountable Odds (53, p. 874).

References

1. Frank, A. W. (1991). *At the will of the body: Reflections on illness.* Boston: Houghton Mifflin.
2. American Cancer Society. (1994). *Cancer facts & figures—1994.* Atlanta, 1.
3. Bush, N. E., Haberman, M. R., Donaldson, G., & Sullivan, K. M. (1995). Quality of life of 125 adults surviving 6–18 years after bone marrow transplantation. *Social Science and Medicine, 40,* 479–490.
4. Gottheil, E., McGurn, W. C., & Pollack, O. (1979). Awareness and disengagement in cancer patients. *American Journal of Psychiatry, 136,* 632–636.
5. Haberman, M. R. (1995). The meaning of cancer therapy: Bone marrow transplantation as an exemplar of therapy. *Seminars in Oncology Nursing, 11,* 23–31.
6. Mullan, F. (1985). Seasons of survival: Reflections of a physician with cancer. *New England Journal of Medicine, 313,* 270–273.
7. Mages, N. L., & Mendelsohn, G. A. (1980). Effects of cancer on patient's lives: A personological approach. In G. C. Stone, F. Cohen, & N. E. Adler (Eds.), *Health psychology—A handbook.* (pp. 255–284). San Francisco: Jossey-Bass.
8. Leigh, S., Boyle, D. M., Loescher, L. J., & Hoffman, B. (1993). Psychosocial issues of long-term survival from adult cancer. In S. L. Groenwald, M. H. Frogge, M. Goodman, & C. H. Yarbo (Eds.), *Cancer nursing. Principles and practice.* (3rd. ed.), (pp. 484–495). Boston: Jones and Bartlett.
9. Leigh, S. (1994, Summer). Our presence is vital. In E. Hermanson (Ed.), *Networker, 8,* (p. 2). Silver Spring: National Coalition for Cancer Survivorship.
10. Weisman, A. D., & Worden, J. W. (1976-1977). The existential plight in cancer: Significance of the first 100 days. *International Journal of Psychiatry in Medicine, 7,* 1–15.
11. Maher, E. L. (1982). Anomic aspects of recovery from cancer. *Social Science and Medicine, 16,* 907–912.
12. Fletcher, D. M. (1992). Unconventional cancer treatments: Professional, legal, and ethical issues. *Oncology Nursing Forum, 19,* 1351–1354.
13. Montbriand, M. J. (1993). Freedom of choice: An issue concerning alternate therapies chosen by patients with cancer. *Oncology Nursing Forum, 20,* 1195–1201.
14. Roud, P. C. (1987). Psychosocial variables associated with the exceptional

survival of patients with advanced malignant disease. *Journal of the National Medical Association, 79,* 97–102.

15. Shanfield, S. B. (1980). On surviving cancer: Psychological considerations. *Comprehensive Psychiatry, 21,* 128–134.
16. Eakes, G. G. (1993). Chronic sorrow: A response to living with cancer. *Oncology Nursing Forum, 20,* 1327–1334.
17. Hassey-Dow, K. (1990). The enduring seasons in survival. *Oncology Nursing Forum, 17,* 511–516.
18. Holland, J. C. (1989). Clinical course of cancer. In Holland, J. C., & J. H. Rowland (Eds.), *Handbook of psychooncology: Psychological care of the patient with cancer* (pp. 75–100). New York: Oxford University Press.
19. Fiore, N. A. (1979, February 8). Fighting cancer—one patient's perspective. *New England Journal of Medicine, 300,* 284–289.
20. Welch-McCaffrey, D., Hoffman, B., Leigh, S. A., Loescher, L. J., & Meyskens, F. L., Jr. (1989). Surviving adult cancers. Part 2. Psychosocial implications. *Annals of Internal Medicine, 111,* 517–524.
21. Parkes, C. M. (1971). Psychosocial transitions: A field for study. *Social Science and Medicine, 5,* 101–115.
22. Fiore, N. A. (1984). *The road back to health: Coping with the emotional side of cancer.* Toronto: Bantam.
23. Taylor, S. (1983, November). Adjustments to threatening events: A theory of cognitive adaptation. *American Psychology,* 1161–1173.
24. Johnston-Taylor, E. (1993). Factors associated with meaning of life among people with recurrent cancer. *Oncology Nursing Forum, 20,* 1399–1405.
25. Loescher, L. J., Clark, L., Atwood, J. R., Leigh, S., & Lamb, G. (1990). The impact of the cancer experience on long-term survivors. *Oncology Nursing Forum, 17,* 223–229.
26. Mood, D. W. (1991). The diagnosis of cancer: A life transformation. In S. B. Baird, R. McCorkle, & M. Grant (Eds.), *Cancer nursing: A comprehensive textbook.* (pp. 219–234). Philadelphia: W. B. Saunders.
27. Haberman, M. R. (1987). Living with leukemia: The personal meaning attributed to illness and treatment by adults undergoing a bone marrow transplantation. (Doctoral dissertation, University of Washington, 1987). *Dissertation Abstracts International, 48/03-B,* p. 703.
28. Lewis, F. M. (1982). Experienced personal control and quality of life in late-stage cancer patients. *Nursing Research, 31,* 113–119.
29. Lewis, F. M., Haberman, M. R., & Wallhagen, M. (1986). How late-stage adult cancer patients experience control. *Journal of Psychosocial Oncology, 4,* 27–42.
30. Cella, D. F. (1987). Cancer survival: Psychosocial and public issues. *Cancer Investigation, 5,* 59–67.
31. Mahon, S. M. (1991). Managing the psychosocial consequences of cancer recurrence: Implications for nurses. *Oncology Nursing Forum, 18,* 577–583.
32. Schmale, A. H. (1976). Psychological reactions to recurrences, metastases, or disseminated cancer. *International Journal of Radiation, Oncology, Biology, and Physics, 1,* 515–520.
33. Cella, D. F., Mahon, S. M., & Donovan, M. I. (1990, Spring). Cancer recurrence as a traumatic event. *Behavioral Medicine,* pp. 15–22.
34. Weisman, A. D., & Worden, J. W. (1986). The emotional impact of recurrent cancer. *Journal of Psychosocial Oncology, 3,* 5–16.
35. Mullan, R. (1984). Re-entry: The educational needs of the cancer survivor. *Health Education Quarterly, 10*(Suppl.), 88–94.
36. United States Department of Health and Human Services. (1987). *When cancer recurs: Meeting the challenge again.* (NIH Publication No. 87–2709).

37. Haberman, M. R., Bush, N., Young, K., & Sullivan, K. M. (1993). Quality of life of adult long-term survivors of bone marrow transplantation: A qualitative analysis of narrative data. *Oncology Nursing Forum, 20,* 1545–1553.
38. Smith, K., & Lesko, L. M. (1988, January). Psychosocial problems in cancer survivorship. *Oncology,* pp. 33–44.
39. Hoffman, B. (1989). Cancer survivors at work: Job problems and illegal discrimination. *Oncology Nursing Forum, 16,* 39–43.
40. Tross, S., & Holland, J. C. (1989). Psychological sequelae in cancer survivors. In Holland, J. C., & J. H. Rowland (Eds.), *Handbook of psychooncology: Psychological care of the patient with cancer.* (pp. 101–116). New York: Oxford University Press.
41. Ferrell, B., Grant, M., Schmidt, G. M., Rhiner, M., Whitehead, C., Fonbuena, P., & Forman, S. J. (1992). The meaning of quality of life for bone marrow transplant survivors. Part 2. Improving quality of life for bone marrow transplant survivors. *Cancer Nursing, 15,* 247–253.
42. Haberman, M. R., Woods, N. F., & Packard, N. J. (1990). Demands of chronic illness: Reliability and validity assessment of a demands-of-illness inventory. *Holistic Nursing Practice, 5,* 25–35.
43. Packard, N. J., Haberman, M. R., Woods, N. F., & Yates, B. C. (1991). Demands of illness among chronically ill women. *Western Journal of Nursing Research, 13,* 434–457.
44. Woods, N. F., Haberman, M. R., & Packard, N. J. (1993). Demands of illness and individual dyadic, and family adaptation in chronic illness. *Western Journal of Nursing Research, 15,* 10–30.
45. Haney, C. A. (1984). Psychosocial factors in the management of patient with cancer. In C. L. Cooper (Ed.), *Psychosocial stress and cancer.* (pp. 201–227). New York: John Wiley & Sons.
46. Wortman, C. B., & Dunkel-Schetter, C. (1979). Interpersonal relationships and cancer: A theoretical analysis. *Journal of Social Issues, 35,* 120–155.
47. Spiegel, D. (1993). Psychosocial intervention in cancer. *Journal of the National Cancer Institute, 85,* 1198–1205.
48. National Coalition for Cancer Survivorship, (1994, Summer). *Networker, 8,* Silver Spring.
49. Stewart, S. (1994, September). *BMT Newsletter.* Highland Park.
50. United States Department of Health and Human Services. (1990, July). *Facing forward: A guide for cancer survivors.* (NIH Publication No. 90-2424).
51. Morra, M., & Potts, E. (1990). *Triumph, Getting back to normal when you have cancer.* New York: Avon Books.
52. Broder, S. (1994). Cancer research today. *Coping, 9,* 11–12.
53. Bushkin, E. (1993). Signposts of survivorship. *Oncology Nursing Forum, 20,* 869–875.

Part Three

Professional Perspectives

Unendurable Pain

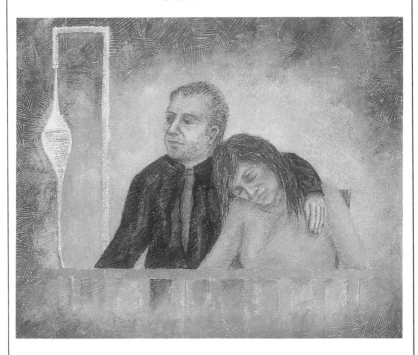

Chapter 6

Physician's Perspective on Suffering

Robert Dunlop, MD

St. Christopher's Hospice

THE TWENTIETH CENTURY has seen an exponential increase in the number of investigations and treatments for disease. Cures are now possible for some illnesses, life expectancy can be extended for others, and even when it is not possible to alter prognosis there is a high likelihood that the pathophysiology of the condition will be well understood.

With these advances in medical science has come the prospect of new life for many patients. When this happens, the gratitude of the patient and family will be profuse. Physicians enjoy receiving thanks for a successful resuscitation or a life-saving operation. Many medical institutions have been founded or supported by financial contributions from grateful patients and families.

For the physicians, there is the added exhilaration of battling with and then overcoming disease. The management of an acute trauma victim with multiple injuries produces an adrenalin rush. The intellectual challenge is exemplified by the intensive care setting. There, medical staff have to interpret a constant stream of information and then fine-tune the response. At times the work can be routine, but life-threatening complications are always likely and must be preempted if possible. It can be immensely rewarding to see the patient "walk out" and know that death has been cheated.

Despite these advances, it is clear that the medical profession has not adequately addressed some of the major problems experienced by patients. One example was highlighted in a recent paper published by Cleeland et al. (3). The Eastern Cooperative Oncology Group (ECOG) reviewed the incidence of pain in patients undergoing anticancer treatments. It is particularly distressing that patients were experiencing severe pain despite the fact that the management of cancer pain is well documented. Many patients were receiving inadequate pain treatments. The study also showed that nonmedical factors were influencing pain management: young women and patients from ethnic minorities were more likely to have uncontrolled pain.

The needs of families are also often not being considered, particularly in the acute hospital setting. Hockley et al. (6) carried out a prospective survey of patients with an estimated prognosis of less than three months. Relatives were also interviewed using a semistructured format and a mood adjective checklist. The relatives described a variety of problems that had not been addressed. The most common physical symptom was fatigue, exacerbated by a lack of community support in many cases. Some relatives even became physically ill from the burden of care. Psychological distress included depression, fear, and anxiety. These emotions were associated with unrelieved patient symptoms including pain. When the patient could not be cared for at home, the relative was often left feeling very guilty. When the patient died, relatives were left to cope with these unresolved feelings as well as the impact of the loss.

Health professionals contributed to relatives' distress by not giving them adequate information or by giving conflicting statements about prognosis. Most relatives had to form their own impressions of how ill the patients were. One third of relatives had never spoken to a physician during the admission, and half were given inadequate information. Relatives were usually too afraid to "bother" health professionals with their need for more information.

This chapter will examine why these serious deficits in care exist, using the perspectives of the physician as a person and the physician as a professional. The concept of suffering will be briefly explored, and an historical perspective on how physicians have dealt with suffering will be offered. The chapter will conclude with some observations on how physicians can care for the suffering patient and some recommendations for training.

What Is Suffering?

Most people, including many physicians, have come to think of suffering as an unpleasant but transient reaction to an acute event, such as "suffering from a headache." The true meaning of the word has been diluted by everyday use in phrases like "suffering a setback." Cassel (2) defined suffering as "the state of severe distress associated with events that threaten the intactness of the person." This definition emphasizes the intensely personal nature of suffering and the very serious threat to the person's integrity. The events that cause suffering are perceived as being out of control, with no forseeable end, beyond help.

A variety of causes may produce this level of distress, many of which fall outside the remit of the physician. However, ill health whether real or perceived is a potent cause of suffering. Furthermore, the physical and psychological manifestations of severe distress from nonmedical causes may also prompt the person or their relatives to seek attention from a physician. Treatment for medical conditions can cause suffering, and this prospect real or imagined may cause patients to make decisions contrary to the advice of the physician. It therefore behooves all physicians to have an understanding of suffering.

In the introduction to this chapter, mention was made of patients experiencing unrelieved cancer pain. Not all patients will "suffer" from pain. The prospect of successful anticancer treatment may override any sense that the pain will continue or escalate. Occasionally, a patient will be more distressed by the pain treatment than the pain itself. Fears about the use of morphine abound in the lay as well as the professional communities. The fears that morphine will cause addiction, premature death, uncontrolled pain in the terminal phase, or intellectual obtundation have no basis in reality. Rarely, the pain will serve a positive purpose, for example the expiation of guilt associated with some major traumatic event in the person's past unrelated to the cancer. None of these examples are reasons for not taking pain seriously. They serve to underline the need for a comprehensive assessment of pain.

For most patients, the diagnosis of cancer causes distress about the loss of future opportunities, the loss of dignity, the loss of relationships, and the sense of being a burden. This distress will be exacerbated by the physical effects of pain such as pain intensity and loss of sleep, and the considerable psychosocial effects. For these reasons, cancer pain can be considered as an indicator of suffering, and the experiences of cancer pain patients can be used as a model for understanding how physicians respond to suffering.

Case Study

Mrs. O. was 72 years old when her laryngeal carcinoma was diagnosed. The primary lesion had invaded local tissues and a laryngectomy was required. A traheo-esophageal fistula was created enabling her to speak by means of a valve. Radiotherapy was given after the surgery. For two years post-surgery, she led an active life. Then her husband was struck down by a car when he was crossing the road. He sustained a severe head injury resulting in memory loss and disturbed behavior. Mrs. O. could not look after him at home. He had to be admitted to a nursing home. Mrs. O. blamed herself for not coping and she became very depressed.

Just after her husband was admitted to the nursing home, Mrs. O. began to experience low thoracic back pain. There were no abnormal physical findings. Because of her nervous disposition, Mrs. O. was "reassured." Her pain continued, increasing in severity.

After two months, she was reviewed again. She was now taking regular acetaminophen combined with a weak opioid for the back pain. A 1.5cm lump was now palpable over the spinous process of the tenth thoracic vertebra. The lump was exquisitely tender, as was the surrounding skin over a radius of more than 30cm. She would cry out and flinch even before the skin was touched. It was also apparent that the laryngeal carcinoma had recurred at the tracheostomy stoma. The 1cm malignant ulcer was not causing symptoms.

The radiotherapist became concerned about the obvious recurrence. A repeat course of radiotherapy was prescribed, dose-adjusted to take into account the previous treatment. With regard to Mrs. O.'s pain, the radiotherapist was very dismissive. An x-ray of the spine only showed "minor degenerative changes." Mrs. O.'s reaction to the pain was labelled as "histrionic" but morphine was prescribed as a concessionary measure. The presence of the subcutaneous lump was ignored, despite the fact that it was obviously the cause of the tenderness.

Mrs. O.'s pain continued. More importantly, her distress was escalating rapidly. The pain seemed out of control, there was no diagnosis, and Mrs. O. felt that she was about to die at any moment. She could not sleep at night and her agitation during the day was so upsetting to the family that they could not support her at home. Mrs. O. was very aware of their anguish, which only served to feed her own suffering.

Eventually, Mrs. O. was admitted to a hospice inpatient unit. The pain was diagnosed as superficial somatic pain caused by a subcutaneous metastasis. Topical local anaesthetic cream and nonsteroidal anti-inflammatory tablets were used to gain control of the pain. Mrs. O's agitated depression was treated with a combination of an antidepressant and counselling. Her family were given time to express their fears and concerns as well.

Mrs. O. visited the radiotherapist again just after she was discharged home. She was referred for consideration of radiotherapy to the subcutaneous lump which had grown to over 5cm in diameter. Even though several other painful subcutaneous lumps had appeared, the radiotherapist could not back down from the his previous diagnosis. Mrs. O. and her family were told that there was no evidence of cancer. Fortunately, they were now able to cope with this behavior. The family continued to care for Mrs. O. at home, effectively controlling her pain, until she died. One can only shudder at the thought of what might have happened if the hospice had not been involved.

A Brief Historical Perspective

This chapter began by emphasizing the positive value of technological advances in medicine. Medical oncology, for example, has benefited enormously from these advances: cytogenetics has increased the understanding of cancer behavior, new biopsy and pathology techniques have improved diagnostic accuracy, CT and MRI scanners have revolutionized staging and the assessment of treatment response, and there is a plethora of drug regimens for treatment. Some people point to these advances as being a major cause for the problems in cancer pain management exposed by the ECOG study. It is as if medical oncologists have become blinded by the new technologies and treatments, blinded so that the cancer process rather than the patient has become the focus. This perspective harkens back to a romantic notion of medical practice in the pre-antibiotic era. Several paintings portray the family physician sitting at the bedside of a young patient perhaps wracked by the fever and delerium of a pneumococcal pneumonia. A life would be in the balance but the physician could only minister to the nonmedical needs of the family, providing support by visiting regularly and succor by well-chosen words of advice and comfort.

Undoubtedly there were many physicians who were practiced in the art of medicine in those times, just as there are today. But history records that the inadequacies in medical care for patients with incurable diseases long preceded the emergence of the Age of Technology. The earliest history of St. Bartholomew's Hospital, founded in London in 1124 and still the oldest mediaeval hospital in England surviving on its original site, provides some interesting insights.

Like most mediaeval hospitals, St. Bartholomew's was established by a religious order to care for the sick poor. Even though the range of medical treatments was minimal, the emphasis was quickly shifted from care to cure. Relics of the cross were used to effect miraculous cures. By the 16th century, this emphasis had become so significant that it was written into the job description for the surgeons. At a time when anaesthesia did not exist and few operations were possible, the role of the surgeon included defining who was curable and who was incurable so that incurable patients could be kept out of the hospital.

In the 17th century, the Great Plague swept across Europe. The hospital records revealed that the physicians retreated into the country and abandoned the care of patients to the matron and apothecary. During the next 200 years, physicians such as Parkinson and Pott helped characterize diseases and increase the range of therapies. However, the lack of attention to the needs of the dying eventually led to the establishment of religious institutions such as St. Joseph's Hospice, which was built in 1904 only two miles from St Bartholomew's Hospital. These institutions were the forerunners of the Modern Hospice Movement founded in 1967 by Dame Cicely Saunders.

The preoccupation of medical practice with cure and the associated marginalization of suffering terminally ill patients clearly preceded the advent of high technology medicine. Other factors, both personal and professional, must be involved in perpetuating this situation. Some of these factors will be explored in the next section.

The Physician as a Person

When considering the physician's perspective on suffering, it is important to acknowledge that he or she is first and foremost an individual within society. Most people have a fear of death that operates at a subconscious level. Solomon et al. (10) have investigated this fear using a number of elaborate experiments. Subjects exposed to videos emphasizing death became more intolerant of situations and people who differed from the subjects' cultural norms and expectations. This same reaction occurs when people are confronted with unrelieved suffering.

In one of the oldest discourses on suffering, Job has virtually everything taken away from him: his material possessions, his family, and his health. The intolerance of Job's "comforters" is illustrated by their various responses. They try to give him advice (for example, Job, Chapters 4 and 5) which only serves to show how they have failed to understand his suffering. Job's despair increases which causes the friends to become angry with him (Job 11: 2–3). Eventually they begin to take Job's comments personally (Job 20: 2–3) which leads them to try to make Job feel that his suffering is his fault (Job, Chapter 22).

Socially, physicians tend to be drawn from "successful" families who can afford the cost of the higher education necessary to enter medical school. Even with scholarships and other financial awards, medical training remains very expensive. These factors discourage candidates who are not white middle- or upperclass. Consequently, most physicians have little understanding of the needs of ethnic minorities and patients from lower socioeconomic backgrounds. This is reflected in the greater dissatisfaction expressed by black patients about the qualitative ways that their physicians treat them (1).

Medical students and newly graduated physicians are likely to have a limited personal experience of suffering. People usually enter medical school in their late teens or early twenties. They will have been consistently successful academically at school. They are unlikely to have experienced a major physical illness; many will still have parents and grandparents living. Not that people embarking on a career in any of the health professions need first-hand experience of illness. Indeed there can be major problems if health professionals base their practice on their past experiences, whether consciously or not, as illustrated by the process of counter-transference. What is needed is the ability to empathize with patients while maintaining a degree of detachment and self-awareness. If used correctly, personal experience may sharpen the empathic process. In the absence of such experience, empathy toward the suffering of others has to be actively taught, along with an awareness of social factors that dull the process.

Observers from other cultures have written about Western societal traits that impede empathy. Latin American theologians have been particularly insightful. Gutierrez (5) first described a theology of liberation, exposing the strategies which prevent people from recognizing and responding to the suffering of the poor. One of the most important strategies is to relabel situations that appear threatening. For example, the poor are often described as "lazy," which then excuses any role that discrimination might play in maintaining poverty. Pharoah's reaction to the plight of the Hebrews in Egypt is used as an example of relabeling (Exodus, Chapter 5).

In the clinical setting, relabeling can be seen with cancer pain patients. Wilkes (11) compared health professionals interpretations of patients' symptoms with that of relatives. He found that physicians significantly under-reported the incidence of pain. Instead, they over-reported that patients were anxious. Relabeling pain as anxiety removes the problem from the realm of medical science and obviates the need to use analgesic drugs. The patient becomes the "problem," not the pain or the physician's inability to control the pain.

The process of relabelling has similarities to the strategies that men have often subconsciously used against women. For example a man will be described as "assertive," a woman as "aggressive." In the past, virtually all physicians were male. Traditionally, men are less likely to acknowledge emotions either in themselves or in others. These traits make it difficult to seek for and recognize suffering in others. Fortunately, the number of women physicians is increasing rapidly and they are having an important impact on the way medicine is practiced.

The Physician as a Professional

Science and technology are an integral part of medicine. The emphasis on the scientific approach begins before entry into medical school; very few students who major in the arts will be accepted. The student of science must learn to be dispassionate, to look for observable, measurable facts, and to arrange these observations into patterns. The medical model perpetuates this process. Diseases are taught as discrete entities comprising specific clinical and other findings. The importance of accurate diagnosis and treatment is stressed throughout the training process; curable diseases must not be missed.

However, few medical schools provide any significant teaching on the concept of the whole person or on the nature of suffering. Thus, when a patient is asked to give a history, the examining physician will usually focus on those elements of the history which support a diagnosis. The embellishments that the patient adds to the story are frequently disregarded even though they contain powerful messages about what the patient is worrying about. Some teaching is offered about communication skills and usually comprises role plays or similar techniques. Teaching about pain control is still very limited.

Most clinical teaching takes place in acute hospitals that are orientated towards diagnosis and cure. Students are less likely to have contact with the chronically ill or the elderly. Although closer contact will be made with other health professionals in the ward settings, the training is uniprofessional. Teamworking will be observed on some services such as pediatrics, but the principles will not be specifically espoused. During their clinical attachments, students are not allowed to say "I don't know" in response to a question from the tutor. This makes it difficult for physicians to acknowledge any deficits in their knowledge and compromises the possibility of multidisciplinary teamwork. When this difficulty is coupled with a lack of teaching on pain control and suffering, it is not surprising that physicians use avoidance strategies such as walking past the room of a dying patient on the ward round.

After qualification, physicians enter into a period of apprenticeship learning, still within the acute hospitals. During this time, the pressure of work is often considerable and will tend to undo any training in communication skills. Physicians have to become adept at using verbal and nonverbal means of minimizing the time taken to admit or review a patient, such as asking very specific questions which are not open-ended, cutting in when a patient drifts off the subject, and using body language which indicates the physician wants to leave (9). These strategies are reinforced by the lack of alternative role models from senior colleagues.

All of the aforementioned constraints on care are compounded by the problems that patients have in expressing their needs. Cultural and class differences will increase these difficulties. Cancer patients have demonstrated a high social desirability, a need to provide responses that please the physician (7). Relatives are rarely able to act as the patient's advocate. Reference has already been made earlier in this chapter to the reasons why this is so.

In summary, physicians have difficulty recognizing and dealing with suffering for a variety of reasons, personal and professional. Most people want to avoid distressing situations that are personally threatening, particularly if they have not been given the knowledge or skills to handle those situations. Personal avoidance techniques such as denial and relabeling are reinforced by professional training. There is already a groundswell for change. Quite apart from the increasing expectations of patients and families, physicians are becoming more aware of these issues. Before examining how the medical management of suffering may be improved, the physician's role in the dealing with suffering will be reviewed.

The Physician's Role in the Management of Suffering

Physicians have an important role with patients who are suffering. Before looking at this role in detail, the value of other health professionals must be acknowledged. The Hospice Movement has emphasized the necessity of multidisciplinary teamworking. Physicians need the personal and professional perspectives available from other disciplines, particularly because patients present different information to physicians. Some physicians have difficulty acknowledging that specialist nurses may know more about pain control for example; professional humility is essential for the best care of patients.

A foremost role of the physician is that of listener. People who are suffering need to have their experiences validated. Too often, their pleas for help have been disregarded, worse still denegrated by comments such as "it is all in the mind," "there is nothing physically wrong," or "pull yourself together." Listening requires a nonjudgmental approach that accepts whatever information the person wants to offer even if that information does not fall easily into a known medical syndrome. Listening also requires time.

Suffering has a significant future component. The sense of a problem continuing unabated causes the most distress. Therefore, history-taking should focus on the patient's fears for the future. A helpful question can be: "What is the worst thing that you think could happen to you?" Patients should be encouraged to describe how they think the illness is affecting and will affect them. Sensitive inquiry along these lines will often reveal dramatic vivid images that may have little basis in medical fact but clearly cause anguish. Patients variously describe cancer as "rotting inside," "about to cause the abdomen to explode" in the case of ascites, or "about to strangle and suffocate" in the case of lung cancer. Because few patients have seen someone die, except on television where death from cancer occurs in actors whose physical appearance does not change, pain is often seen as the harbinger of death.

While patients' comments must be respected, other perspectives should be sought, particularly those of the family. Health professionals who can visit in the home such as home health visitors and social workers can provide helpful insights. A joint meeting with the patient and family can be very useful. Patients often worry about being a burden, but seldom verbalize these fears to their relatives. Openly addressing these worries may resolve some of the suffering.

To be an effective listener, it is necessary to lay aside the need to provide an answer, at least in the early stages. Too often physicians go into "information mode" when confronted with a distressed patient, providing reams of medical jargon intended to reassure the patient. However, the nonverbal message is that the physician cannot handle distress. Just allowing the person to talk will often prove therapeutic. When deep-seated fears are verbalized, they become more concrete, less frightening, and may even dissolve in the telling. Inaccurate attributions such as the fear of dying from pain can be gently corrected, but the effect of reassurance must always be reviewed in the light of the patient's subsequent behaviour.

Suffering often centers on physical symptoms. Physicians have an important role to play in treating these symptoms. There is a vast body of literature about palliating the variety of problems that occur when the disease itself cannot be treated. For example, excellent guidelines have now been published that clearly describe how to assess and treat cancer pain (8).

The treatment of symptoms should not await a diagnosis. However, the role of the physician as a diagnostician is very important. Not only does a diagnosis validate the patient's experience, it also provides a clearer idea of prognosis. Fortunately, the belief that patients should never be told the diagnosis of cancer has been laid to rest. However, about 10 percent of patients will not want to be told; persevering in overcoming their denial will increase suffering.

Another important role of the physician is as advocate. When the physician cannot manage someone's suffering, he or she should not hesitate to ask for advice, not just from other physicians. Patients respect physicians who acknowledge when they are unable to help and refer on appropriately. Other health professionals such as clinical nurse specialists and psychologists have an important role to play. Their counselling skills can help patients and families work through difficult issues. They are often able to teach nonpharmacological strategies for coping with distress, such as relaxation and visualization. Support groups are another important resource. When people come together with a background of shared experiences, they quickly develop an atmosphere of understanding and mutual support. Practical solutions to problems will often be shared. The deep-felt sense of "being in it together" also has a powerful therapeutic effect.

When physicians exercise the roles described above in collaboration with nonphysician colleagues, most patients will regain their sense of control over the future and the intensity of suffering will abate. The relief from fear and uncontrolled symptoms will often allow the remaining months to be very positive: relationships will be mended or strengthened, new opportunities grasped, and a greater sense of self-awareness achieved.

Euthanasia and Physician-Assisted Suicide

Recently, considerable publicity has centered on the use of euthanasia as a treatment for suffering. The debate has been complicated by misunderstandings about what constitutes euthanasia. Most people would accept that life-prolonging treatments such as intravenous nutritional support and ventilation can be withheld when patients with advanced cancer are dying. This is not the same as "active" euthanasia, which is the deliberate termination of a patient's life usually by means of a lethal injection.

Proponents of "active" euthanasia believe that it is a humane way to relieve suffering. In the past, they advocated that physicians should be allowed to administer the lethal injection. Now the role of the physician has been reinterpreted by the concept of physician-assisted suicide. In this role, the physician serves as a technician providing the means by which the patient then self-administers the lethal injection.

The ethical arguments against euthanasia have been clearly established (12). Medical practitioners cannot exercise the diametrically opposed roles of physician and executioner. Patients could not trust their physicians. Suffering patients do occasionally express a wish that death would come more quickly. Further inquiry will reveal that this is a cry for help and understanding. Therefore, they must be able to raise these issues in an atmosphere of trust, not with the shadow of euthanasia clouding the physician–patient relationship.

Euthanasia is practiced in the Netherlands, although it has not been legalized. Pro-euthanasia lobbyists see this as an enlightened approach. However, the Netherlands has very few hospice services (13). Furthermore, despite having the most liberal laws for opioid prescribing, the Netherlands also has one of the lowest rates of morphine usage in Europe. Patients need greater access to good palliative care so that they can receive help. Physicians need to recognize that suffering can be relieved by other means. Otherwise, they will be drawn by default into a situation where euthanasia becomes accepted practice.

Rarely, some cancer patients become extremely distressed when they are dying. These patients have often used high levels of denial to maintain a sense of normality. When the cancer finally renders them too weak to get about, they loose the mental energy necessary to maintain the denial. Physicians often fail to recognize the significance of the ensuing extreme agitation which requires urgent treatment. Sedation may be necessary to prevent the distress escalating and to achieve the relaxed state that normally characterizes dying. This can be achieved by titration with subcutaneous midazolam, usually in 10mg increments at fifteen minute intervals followed by a continuous infusion. Death is not hastened but the horror of total pain is avoided.

Facilitating the Physician's Role in Managing Suffering

If the medical management of suffering is to be improved, the factors which prevent physicians realizing their full potential must be addressed. This must begin at the societal level. Pressures for change are increasing. Not only do lay people have higher expectations of medical care but also the broader issues of sexism and racism are being undermined. These pressures have an effect on potential physicians as well as practicing physicians.

The teaching of medical students must deliberately challenge impediments to good practice. Students should be exposed to other cultures, ideas about health, and other nonhospital examples of care such as hospices. This can be done with speakers from patient groups, ethnic minorities, religious communities, etc. The principles of lateral thinking should be taught. Wherever possible, multiprofessional teaching should be encouraged, along with assignments that demand group working to counterbalance the emphasis on individual learning and achievement. Teaching about communication skills and the concepts of transference must be increased.

At all levels of medical practice, teaching should be available about suffering, symptom control, and palliative care. Didactic teaching is the easiest option but is only of limited value. Physicians learn more by example from good role models, such as specialist multidisciplinary palliative care teams within the hospital setting (4). The process of achieving change is very difficult. Although physicians may be reluctant at first, change can and does happen.

Conclusion

Suffering is an age-old facet of human experience. Physicians have an important role to play in the management of suffering, but a variety of factors have conspired over many centuries to make it difficult for physicians to fulfill this role. The suffering patient provides a challenge that demands a high level of personal as well as professional commitment. Seeing out this challenge by helping someone regain control of life can be immensely rewarding and more than compensates for the cost.

References

1. Blendon, R. J., Aiken, L. H., Freeman, H. E., et al. (1989). Access to medical care for black and white Americans. *JAMA, 261*, 278–281.
2. Cassel, E. (1982). The nature of suffering and the goals of medicine. *New England Journal of Medicine, 306*, 639–645.
3. Cleeland, C. S., Gonin, R., Hatfield, A. K., et al. (1994). Pain and pain treatment in outpatients with metastatic cancer: The Eastern Co-operative Oncology Group's Outpatient Pain Study. *New England Journal of Medicine, 330*, 592–596.
4. Dunlop, R. J., & Hockley, J. M. (Eds). (1990) Terminal care support teams: The hospital/hospice interface. London: Oxford Press.
5. Gutierrez, G. (1993). A theology of liberation. New York: Orbis.
6. Hockley, J. M., Dunlop, R. J., & Davies, R. J. (1988). Survey of distressing symptoms in dying patients and their families in hospital and the response to a symptom control team. *British Medical Journal, 296*, 1715–1717.
7. Hurny, C., Piasetsky, E., Bagin, R., et al. (1987). High social desirability in cancer patients being treated for advanced colorectal or bladder cancer: Eventual impact on the assessment of quality of life. *Journal of Psychosocial Oncology, 5*, 19–29.
8. Jacox, A. K., Carr, D. B., & Payne, R., et al. (1994). Management of cancer pain: Clinical practice guidelines No. 9. Rockville, Md.: Agency for Health Care Policy and Research. AHCPR publication no. 94–0592.
9. Macguire, P. (1985). Barriers to psychological care of the dying. *British Medical Journal, 291*, 1711–1713.
10. Solomon, S., Greenberg, J., & Pyszczynski, T. (1991). A terror management theory of social behaviour: The psychological functions of self-esteem and cultural worldviews. Advances in *Experimental Social Psychology, 24*, 93–159.
11. Wilkes, E. Dying now. (1984). *Lancet, 1*, 950–952.
12. Wilkinson, J. (1990). The ethics of euthanasia. *Palliative Medicine, 4*, 81–86.
13. Zylicz, Z. (1993). The story behind the blank spot. *American Journal of Hospice and Palliative Care, 10*, 30–34.

Chapter 7

Theological Perspectives

Father Robert Smith

Religion and Suffering

Religious beliefs and practices touch upon the most fundamental human experiences. The defining moments of our lives, such as birth, marriage, illness or dying, and the emotions and meanings we seek in them, provide the central contents of the great religious traditions. The range and variety of the religious responses to these experiences are enormous. Contained within the great traditions are some of the most profound insights and most creative accomplishments of the human spirit. Among the complex experiences which probe and test human life and its religious interpretations, suffering plays a defining role. For individual people, and for the religious traditions themselves, the confrontation with suffering is a crucial test of their truth and authenticity, the central path to their deepest roots and self-understanding.

Before initiating a discussion of religious responses to suffering, it may be helpful to emphasize the religious roots of our duty to relieve pain. Common to all religious traditions is an acknowledgment of the primary place in human life of compassion and solidarity. These two religious values play an essential role in motivating effective pain treatment. A truly compassionate health care giver will bring to the encounter with patients a habit of trusting and believing, the attentive understanding, and the empathy which play an essential part in asking about and responding to the experience of pain. Furthermore, the religious ideal of the person with compassion for others, together with a sense of solidarity with the needy and marginal, provide motivations that can sustain the care giver in the day-to-day fidelity to the difficult task of pain management. Finally, religious experience creates a sense of community, which can overcome our natural impulse to isolate the person in pain and to distance ourselves from the threat of pain. Within religious experience itself, the control of pain also plays a very important part in the task of helping people to avoid discouragement or even despair. In fidelity to their own traditions, religious communities should be active partners in contemporary efforts to establish throughout the health care system effective and regular treatment of all forms of pain.

Assumptions

In order to discuss the religious response to suffering in the context of contemporary health care, it will help 1) to distinguish suffering from pain, 2) to clarify the relationship between health care and spiritual care, and 3) to justify a general discussion of religion and suffering that necessarily neglects the particular understandings of the several traditions.

1. In ordinary usage, "suffering" and "pain" are often used interchangeably, but for clarity the two terms will be distinguished and the focus will be on religious responses to suffering. Pain and suffering are not identical, and, though in certain forms of terminal and chronic illness they are mutually present and interactive, there are many instances in which one exists without the other. One of the best-known definitions of sufferng is that given by Dr. Eric Cassell: ". . . the state of severe distress associated with events that threaten the intactness of the person."[1]

    Sometimes pain is the signal of the presence of such a threat to continued personal wholeness, and so the occasion for suffering. The suffering itself, however, can continue even when the pain is appropriately controlled. Sometimes chronic pain, even though not life-threatening, is itself a cause of a crisis of personal disintegration. Since suffering has to do with a personal understanding of the meanings of the various dimensions of the self (physical, psychological, and spiritual) and their interrelationships, the presence of suffering cannot be observed from the outside. We can learn of the suffering of others only by attention to the ways in which they express an awareness of such personal wholeness and of threats to its continuance.

2. Illness and its treatment are so urgent and often so dramatic in the lives of people—both the sick and those who care for them—that they risk becoming all-absorbing, reducing all other aspects of our lives to being dimensions of health care. This is particularly dangerous when it is the religious life of the patient that is so affected. Being ill and caring for the ill are moments in a larger human life and experience. Religious beliefs and religious practices are concerned with the whole of

---

[1]Cassell, E. (1991). *The meaning of suffering.* (p. 53). New York: Oxford University Press.

the person's existence; and while spiritual care is rightly integrated into holistic medicine, it is a distortion to see religion as merely an ancillary therapeutic aid. The questions raised by the presence of suffering and our responses to it go beyond the limits of medical therapy. They are considered in literature, the arts and philosophy, and they are lived by ordinary people and creative geniuses in the religious life of humankind.

3. Lastly, we must acknowledge the necessarily schematic and superficial character of this treatment of religion and suffering. There is no single reality that is "religion" or "religious belief," nor is there a common denominator for the rich and complex religious responses to the reality and extent of human suffering. It is not possible here to give even a summary expression of the theological treatments of suffering in the religions to which patients might belong. When and if such questions arise, a referral to an appropriate chaplain or other religious expert should be made. The following discussion will trace some of the places where health care providers might find themselves in the presence of a patient's suffering and of religious responses to that suffering.

Dimensions of Religious Life

In all religious life—whether of individuals or of communities—there are three dimensions that exist in different forms and with differing intensities across various cultures and at each stage of an individual's life. When we are thinking about the religious life, it is helpful to organize our reflections under these three headings: religious life has an intellectual dimension, an ethical dimension, and an experiential dimension. The intellectual dimension can range from highly sophisticated theological and literary expressions to simple stories and folk beliefs. It can exist as strong and firm convictions about the meaning of things or as a searching and questioning struggle to discover such meaning. The ethical dimension of religion—often taking intense form in prophetic voices such as those of Gandhi and Martin Luther King in our own era—shapes both individual lives and institutional patterns in all societies. It often appears in sickness either as a felt obligation to serve the ill or as a challenge for the ill person to respond to sickness with trust and hope. The experiential dimension of religion occurs both in individual experience and in communal experience. For individuals such experiences range from a sense of wholeness and transcendence in the presence of nature, through private prayer and meditation, to extraordinary mystical experiences. Communal religious experience is most frequently organized in formal ritual and worship.

Intellectual Dimension

At the heart of the religious response to suffering is the search for meaning. In fact, the realization of some transcendent meaning which connects the suffering person to some other and greater reality is the source of religious healing—the deliverance from the threat of meaninglessness raised by illness and pain. Such religious deliverance from suffering can exist in the face of continued pain, and even frequently in the face of death. There is a vast literature expressing the search for such meaning and the ways, in the different traditions, in which it may be found. There are, first of all, the scriptures proper to each tradition, and there are as well both ancient and contemporary works ranging from the simple to the very sophisticated. To explore this literature is to live within some of the greatest accomplishments of human genius, and, for health care workers, to glimpse the significance and depth of the work they do every day.

The search for such transcendent meaning in human suffering has always involved great struggle. We think immediately in the Western traditions of the Book of Job, of the sufferings of Jesus, and in the East of the long search for enlightenment of Gotama. For the most part, and in most sickness, such healing insight is not a fixed possession but a peace sustained by love and hope and faithful companionship. One of the geat privileges of those who work in health care is to be the witness to these profound human experiences. Even for health care providers who are not religious themselves, acquaintance with the classic religious literature can provide an appreciation of the human dimensions of pain and illness which can be obscured by the demands and limitations of technical therapy. It can also give a professionally enriching insight into the work of chaplains and others who search with the ill for religious meaning and transcendence.

Ethical Dimension

For the sufferer, the ethical dimension of religious life often occurs as a series of questions about how to respond to the threat of personal disintegration. Suffering can be seen as a test of moral fiber and virtue, as a temptation through which one must pass in order to maintain fidelity to God, as an occasion of personal transformation, and often as a test of the truth and worth of one's previous religious commitments. It is evident that these moral dimensions of suffering touch the most personal and profound levels of each patient's life. They, therefore, require great delicacy and respect on the part of caregivers, especially since the patients' responses can sometimes offend our own deeply felt moral convictions. From a religious perspective, these moral struggles are real tests, and can involve real failures. This is a perspective different from that of therapeutic support proper to the psychological dimension of patient care. In a pluralistic secular environment, indeed in the pluralistic religious environment in which we live, dealing with this moral aspect of religious belief and practice requires wisdom and an understanding informed by attentive communication. Helping people to sort out for themselves what is authentic and inauthentic in their own responses, what the demands and wisdom of their religious tradition might really be are skills necessary in anyone who intends to involve himself or herself in the moral struggles of those who suffer.

One of the most troubling and frequently expressed moral understandings of suffering explains it as a punishment imposed by God for past faults. This can be particularly dangerous when it is an attitude about the suffering of others, and used as a reason not to do what is needed to relieve their suffering or pain. There is no support for such attitudes in the major religious traditions, although they are sometimes cited as a basis of such personal beliefs. The relationship between pain and moral evil is discussed within the scriptures and among the thinkers in all religious traditions, and, over the centuries, a great variety of answers have been given to the questions raised. In the course of these discussions some traditions have included theories of retribution, of punishment as a just restoration of balance, or as a purification of the sinner. Certainly the fact of innocent suffering—as exemplified in the Book of Job and the story of Jesus—provides a major focus of reflection, and one of the principal pathways into to the heart of religious belief and practice. The possible meanings of pain are so many, and the reality of suffering in a person's life so complex, that reducing all of this to a single cause as punishment seems simplistic. It may be psychologically understandable as a first reaction, but it betrays the human richness of religious beliefs, and seems to most religious people to imply a grotesque misunderstanding of God.

Most spiritual writers speak of suffering as a school of learning, correction, or advancing wisdom. It follows that the sufferer's own understanding and interpretation of his or her suffering might change over time, and we should not assume that first interpretations are fixed and changeless. Also, those who are witnesses to the suffering of others must guard against imposing interpretations on them. When everything has been done to assure relief of pain, the principal attitude of caregivers is best one of sympathetic attention. We are at school to those in the school of suffering. The very important religious task is to penetrate the isolation of suffering with genuine and faithful companionship.

Experiential Dimension

The experiential dimension of religion touches on many aspects of suffering and pain. The experience of suffering is a kind of temptation, something that the person must pass through, and in passing through it, will be changed for better or worse. The reality of suffering puts into question one's own life, the meaning of the lives of others, and of the relationship of these lives to one another and to God. This dangerous journey into the mystery of suffering is one of the constant themes of religious scriptures, and the practical wisdom literature of the various traditions contains the insights and advice gained over centuries of human experience. As we pointed out at the beginning of this chapter, suffering arises from the threat to my personal integrity or existence. Since all of us face death, it is impossible to have a human life that would be without suffering, at least not one lived at any depth.

There is another less common, but extremely important, religious experience of suffering which finds in suffering a privileged access to transcendence and a unique and redemptive relation to the lives of other people. As a spiritual ideal, though not a universal obligation, this understanding of the experience of suffering is present in the Christian tradition, and it is here that health care providers might most often encounter it. While it is quite foreign to contemporary cultural ideas, such an experience of suffering, when it occurs authentically, can have remarkable transformative power in the lives of people. Both psychological sophistication and spiritual wisdom and prudence will play a role in accompanying a suffering person in living the experience of suffering in such loving communion with God and others. As with any experience, these religious experiences of suffering occur across a wide range of intensities and forms of expression.

Besides the individual experiences of suffering just discussed, there are the great variety of communal and ritual religious experiences which comfort the sick, offer hope of physical and spiritual healing, and remind the sufferers that they are still connected to communities of life and care. In many hospitals with religious origins, such rituals are part of the ordinary routine. The most commonly known are Christian rituals such as the sharing of the Eucharist, the annointing of the sick, Baptisms of severely ill babies, and various blessings of the dying. In all settings, when it is practically possible and personally acceptable, the professional care giver helps greatly by participating— even as a respectful observer—in the religious rituals and the formal activities of chaplains and other religious representatives.

Afterword

As David Morris demonstrates, suffering and pain are always inter-preted experiences, varying among cultures and individuals.[2] The re-ligious experience of suffering—mediated through religion's own intellectual, ethical, or experiential dimensions—opens the therapeutic medical encounter into very large and richly complex human worlds. The summary provided here necessarily lacks the power and interest which can be found only in the details of each tradition's long struggle with the questions and challenges of human suffering. This chapter provides a framework into which we might place the individual re-sponses to suffering met in the care of the sick, as well as some ways to organize our own reflections and personal questions in the face of this enduring human mystery.

While our culture respects the individual and the individual's world of meaning, its secularism has produced a widespread suspicion of religious belief, or at least a loss of contact with, and understanding

---

[2]Morris, D. (1991). The culture of pain. Berkeley and Los Angles: The University of California Press.

of, traditional religious symbols and experience. At the same time there is both a growing seach for spiritual meaning in life, and a valorization of the cultural pluralism in global human experience. This provides us with a unique opportunity to explore the religious traditions of many people in order to find within them insights and responses to human pain and suffering. How to integrate this human religious inheritance with the rapidly developing science and technology of health care is a challenge which will require the genius and good will of all of us whose privilege it is to be companions to those who suffer. As a first step, we need to realize that illness and the care of the ill take place within a larger human world. While those who care for the ill are in daily contact with profound and revelatory human experiences, they need the richness of attention provided by religious traditions, literature, and the arts in order to integrate these experiences into their own life and to inform the wider culture with their insights. Stories, films, and music can provide us with the language we lack in our culture to express to one another, and so make available to all, an awareness of the depth and value of the human experiences we share.

Across all the range of human experiences of suffering, there is one constant element: the isolation and solitude of the sufferer. Within all the differences of religious understandings and responses to suffering there is one constant for healing: compassionate solidarity. This is not only needed for healing, but it is the root of the development of human wisdom and of the encounter with the Transcendent.

The Christian Traditions

By far the greatest number of religious believers in the United States belong to one of the several Christian traditions, and so it may be a practical help to those who accompany and care for the sick and suffering to speak in some more explicit detail about a Christian experience of suffering. While we will be drawing on the resources of the Catholic tradition, there is a sufficient sharing of beliefs and practices among all Christians to make what we will say to be of general significance.

There is a frequently repeated misunderstanding of Catholic belief that makes suffering a good thing in itself, or views it as a punishment for past faults. Neither of these interpretations has any solid basis in the tradition's image of an infinitely compassionate and forgiving God.

To emphasize expressions of guilt and punishment is to make a religious mistake of concentrating on ourselves rather than on the mystery of God's love in our lives. Whatever helps the sufferer to recognize or reflect on this presence is a most effective aspect of good pastoral care. Most effective is the simple, attentive, and nonjudgmental presence of compassionate believers, whether or not they are official pastoral ministers.

Equally importantly, the Christian faith does not see religion as a way of escaping any of the real dimensions of human experience. It is a way of being human, not a way of escaping human life, or of protecting the believer from human trouble. So the remark often heard "How could this happen to her, when she has lived so faithfully?" is an understandable expression of dismay in the face of human pain, but it is not a response coming from a deep Christian consciousness.

In Christian belief, suffering is a mystery, that is, it is a reality we can never completely grasp or comprehend. Like the mystery of human or divine love, we can experience and understand more and more of the reality of suffering without ever mastering it or exhausting its meaning. When Christians speak of the "mystery" of suffering, they refer, first of all, to the suffering of Christ, which both reveals something of the inner reality of God and is part of the reconciliation of human and divine being. In the second place, this "mystery" expresses a belief that human suffering and pain can be lived through with love. Thus the Christian mystery of suffering is a paradox. The inner drama of suffering and extreme pain is one of isolation and destruction of the self, as we have already said. For Christians this dynamism was reversed in the sufferings of Christ, and his suffering became an act of solidarity and communion. In this, he accomplished the salvation of the world. It is possible, according to the Christian tradition, that some men and women are able to unite their own suffering to that of Christ—and so their suffering becomes a place of communion and love. This is a mysterious and extremely delicate understanding of suffering. It should never be imposed on someone else. Even for those who feel themselves called to live their suffering in solidarity with Christ, out of love there should always be an accompaniment that is prudent and filled with the wisdom of experience and compassion. Thus suffering can become a personal journey of transformation in the lives of individual women and men. Such a mystery is always an invitation to human freedom; it can be entered only by the unforced and conscious choice of the person, and its meanings cannot be described abstractly beforehand.

This is one aspect of the Christian experience of suffering. It is an ideal sometimes reached in the lives of people. Far more common is an experience that is a mixture of success and failure, of faith and doubt. Great pain dominates the lives of people, tending to fix their attention on it and themselves. For this reason alone, Christians should do everything possible to reduce the pain of others, to restore them to themselves. The suffering of others is always an invitation to solidarity. In living out this solidarity in all its complexity, Christians believe that they themselves can encounter the mystery of divine compassion. It is not necessary to idealize the experience of human suffering in order to discover within it the reality of human love and moments of encounter with something that transcends human reality. In fact, the paradox at the heart of the Christian Gospels is the assertion that human failure and human illness can be lived in such a way as to become places of encounter with God. In this sense, suffering is seen as a sort of temptation, that is, an experience in which we live out the possibility of meeting or failing to meet God in our own life, or in the lives of others.

As must by now be evident, there is no simple meaning of suffering in the Christian—or any other—religious tradition. There is certainly a rejection of an extreme contemporary view which holds that suffering is only evil and meaningless. But the communion and solidarity that are the core of the Christian search for meaning in the presence of suffering are not easily described concepts. They will necessarily be filled with the individual particulars and personal life stories of the people involved—both of those who suffer and of those who accompany and care for them. For this reason, communities of support are essential, not only for psychological support but for spiritual and religious support as well.

Two groups of people especially need such communities of spiritual support: the families of those who suffer, and the professional health care givers whose daily work involves them over and over in the suffering of others. For both groups there is need not only for respite, a chance to express the complex feelings that surround prolonged pain and illness and the awareness that one is not unique in these feelings, but also for spiritual insight and companionship in order to integrate these demanding experiences in one's own personal life. The religious pluralism of our culture creates special challenges for such spiritual integration. The key to benefiting from this pluralism is attentive listening, learning to be simply witnesses to the religious journeys of one another. Any group that is mature and open can achieve something valuable in listening to one another. For an individual spiritual journey within a particular tradition, obviously there is needed the guidance of someone wise and experienced in the life of that tradition.

The most dramatic societal issue in which the question of suffering plays a role is the current debate about the acceptability of medically assisted suicide. The fear of "meaningless suffering" is one of the most frequently cited reasons given for approving of this profound societal change. Without attempting a detailed consideration of this complex debate, we can notice that the religious search for solidarity and communion among those who suffer and those who accompany and care for them—as exemplified in the hospice movement—is the key to any rejection of suicide. Such solidarity and communion would not condemn the sufferer to a sense of isolation, abandonment, and hopelessness.

As everyone knows, suffering appears in each human life, sometimes devastatingly; and its questions and challenges lie at the heart of every religious tradition. It can destroy lives and families, and it can deepen and transform them. The religious traditions contain centuries of hard-won wisdom, and their followers should become searchers within themselves, and companions for others, in the inescapable tests of human suffering. What is needed is not pious talk, but ordinary human courage, and the patient willingness to probe the mysteries of human and divine love.

Short Bibliography

To explore the depth and richness of the religious response to suffering, we must study the experience and reflections of particular traditions. The following is a brief and very initial bibliography that will help to locate some contemporary resources among the vast number of books in the theological literature.

General

1. Bowker, J. (1970). *Problems of suffering in the religions of the world.* New York: Cambridge University Press.

In the Christian Tradition

1. Richard, L. (1992). *What are they saying about the theology of suffering?* Mahwah, NJ: Paulist Press.
2. Taylor, M. (Ed.) (1973). *The mystery of suffering and death.* Staten Island, NY: Alba House.
3. Hellwig, M. (1985). *Jesus the compassion of god.* New York: Michael Glazier.
4. Hauerwas, S. (1990). *Naming the silences: God, medicine, and the problem of suffering.* Grand Rapids, MI: Eerdmans.
5. Nouwen, H. (1979). *The wounded healer.* Garden City, NY: Image Books.
6. Beker, J. C. (1987). *Suffering and hope.* Philadelphia: Fortress Press.

In the Jewish Tradition

1. The Jewish way of healing. (1994, Summer). *Reform Judaism Magazine.*
2. Flam, N. (1994, May 27). Reflections toward a theology of illness and healing. *Sh'ma.*
3. *(For further suggestions) The Jewish Healing Center, 141 Alton Ave., San Francisco, CA 94116.*

In the Islamic Tradition

1. Chishti, H. M. *The book of Sufi healing.* Rochester, VT: Inner Tradition International, Ltd.
2. *Sahik AL-Bukhari: The book of medicine,* translated by Dr. Muhamad Muhsin Khan, Dar-Al-Arabia, Beirut, Lebanon.

In the Buddhist Tradition

1. Levine, S. (1989). *Healing into life and death.* Garden City, NY: Doubleday.
2. Levine, S. (1984). *Meeting at the edge: Conversations with the grieving and the dying, the healing and the healed.* Garden City, NY: Doubleday.
3. Sogyal, R. (1994). *The Tibetan book of living and dying.* San Francisco: Harper.

Chapter 8

Coaching and Suffering

The Role of the Nurse
in Helping People Facing Illness

Maman dozed off and woke with a start—her right buttock was hurting. Mme. Gontrand [the nurse] changed her—Maman still complained. I wanted to ring again. "It would still be Mme. Gontrand. She's no good." There was nothing imaginary about Maman's pain; they had exact organic causes . . . they could be soothed by the attentions of Mlle. Parent or Mlle. Martin [nurses]; exactly the same things done by Mme. Gontrand did not ease her. (1, pp. 93–94)

She [the nurse] knew her business—when you are in fear of death, a nurse who knows her business is a pearl beyond price (2, p. 52).

Judith A. Spross, PhD (cand.), RN, OCN, FAAN

Braintree Hospital

Introduction

Patients and families assume that nurses are experts at comforting sufferers. The above two quotations reflect experiences with life-threatening illnesses and illustrate the importance of skilled nursing care in ameliorating suffering. As the first statement points out, actions alone are insufficient to comfort effectively. How nurses are with patients, their interpersonal competence, affects whether patients and families feel comforted. Alleviating suffering, or finding meaning in experiences of suffering, in this author's opinion, depends on intrapersonal and interpersonal qualities nurses bring to their encounters with patients and families; these qualities can be taught and learned. The ability to engage with other human beings as they struggle with suffering is always important; it is especially so when sources of suffering cannot be minimized or eliminated.

Suffering is often used to describe human experiences associated with illness, pain, dying, loss, or grief. Suffering can overwhelm human thought and action and undermine quality of life; suffering can also be positive, serving to uncover meaning, hope, and new possibilities. Sufferers can discover previously untapped courage, wisdom, and personal knowledge that lead to enhanced coping and foster personal growth and self-understanding (3). Although suffering has been mentioned as a focus of nursing care (4) in fact, little research has been done to develop a body of knowledge on the subject (5), (6), (7).

The purpose of this chapter is to offer the reader a nursing perspective on suffering. The author's views on suffering have been informed by extensive experience with patients and families living with cancer and/or pain. The chapter begins with some personal reflections on suffering and the nurse-patient relationship (NPR). Then a selective review of the literature is presented to illustrate the intrapersonal, interpersonal, and social aspects of suffering. Theoretical literature on NPRs is reviewed. The interpersonal nature of comforting those who suffer is further elucidated as a process of coaching. For the most part, the discussion here assumes patients or family members with minimal cognitive impairment. Hospice, critical care, and pediatric nurses know well the nonverbal and behavioral cues that may be indicators of

This work was supported in part by a Boston College University Fellowship and a Doctoral Fellowship from the American Cancer society suffering in preverbal and comatose patients and what interpersonal measures nurses use to comfort them.

Personal Reflections on the Nurse-Patient Relationship and Suffering

As a nursing student 20 years ago, I remember the many process recordings I wrote. These documents were the record of my therapeutic conversations with patients, submitted to faculty, who made notes in the margins, offering feedback—praise or suggestions for improvement. Throughout the curriculum there was an emphasis on interpersonal communications and the therapeutic use of self as a healing modality—these skills became thoroughly integrated into my clinical repertoire. I learned early on that being technically competent was essential but insuffcient. Students were cautioned not to get "overinvolved," to maintain a "professional distance." I understood the message but my work with chronically ill cancer patients led me to rethink this dictum. The notion of distance seemed incongruent with the depth of knowledge and feeling nurses, patients, and families could experience when facing a life-threatening illness, rigorous treatment, or death together. So, as a young nurse, I found it difficult to be a distant nurse. Over the years I began to redefine the notion of distance for myself. It seems that the real message should be to ensure that how nurses feel about patients and families should not undermine their ability to be therapeutic. In addition to challenging the idea of distance, I and other nurses frequently receive calls from physicians to be with patients. They recognize that they cannot provide what the patient or family need—a nurse. More often than not, the request is phrased as: "Mr. Smith needs 'hand-holding'." This is not always meant pejoratively but the label itself diminishes and oversimplifies what I find to be most complex and challenging about nursing. Regardless of the good intentions of the speaker, the view of good or excellent nursing care as "hand-holding" belittles the considerable investment of time, money, energy, and commitments professional nurses make to learn and grow in their careers. When I began to teach direct entry master's students, who were beginning their nursing careers, the drive to understand and articulate these reflections became a quest. This chapter is an opportunity to share some of these reflections.

Snapshots of Suffering

A 50-year-old man is diagnosed with an inoperable brain tumor. He lies awake in the middle of the night, crying, "beside himself," wondering whether his brain will work long enough for him to communicate his deepest thoughts, his love, and his concern to his family. At the same time, he says he doesn't want to cry in front of his grown sons or his partner; his need to be strong and his need to protect his family from "making things worse for them by crying" conflicts with his own need for love and support as he deals with a desperately foreshortened future. He is concerned, too, with the absence of privacy for talking with his family since he is in a two-bed room and is unable to move from the room independently. His mental anguish is accompanied by physical discomforts, particularly the inability to make small adjustments in his position because of left-sided paralysis. In addition to helping the patient change position, the primary interventions are interpersonal: reassuring him that his concerns and tears are normal; eliciting his priorities (talking to his family in private); encouraging him to share his emotions and tears with his family; and making a plan to address his priorities.

A woman, dying of breast cancer, explains to me why she was so "ugly" (mean) to her teen-age daughter when she visited. "I would rather she not come to see me. I cannot bear to see her suffer because I am suffering and I can see it on her face. If I am ugly to her, maybe she won't come to see me, and I can keep her from seeing me like this. But I hate not to see her; I love her and I know I don't have much time" (weeps). Again, the interventions are interpersonal with a focus on acknowledging the distress of the patient (the sufferer) and the daughter (who suffers with and/or because of her mother); what the patient needs from her daughter and what she might be losing by pushing her daughter away; what the nurse can do to find out what the daughter's concerns are; the opportunities that exist for framing the daughter's memories of her mother if the patient is willing to rethink her approach.

A student I taught, after caring for a terminally ill adolescent over the course of a year, noted in his clinical journal, "I was no longer his nurse; I was his friend." With the student's permission, his journal entry was used in class. A long discussion ensued regarding the students' prior experiences with friends and with patients. All of the students could describe situations similar to the one described in the journal entry that sparked the discussion. When brought to consciousness, students were able to describe what was similar and what was different about relationships with patients compared with friends. The nurse-patient relationship isn't friendship but it feels like friendship—if it isn't friendship, what is it?

These snapshots of suffering highlight the interpersonal and intimate nature of nurses' interactions with patients. Travelbee (4) and Martocchio (8) acknowledged the intimate character of the nurse-patient relationship (NPR), and emphasized its importance to establishing authentic and effective therapeutic relationships. They also maintained that nurse-patient relationships are not friendships. However, like the student in the above scenario, three authors (8), (10), (11) offer friendship as an explanation of this intimacy. For a while, after the discussion with the students described above, I tended to characterize the NPR as "one-sided intimacy"—the nurse would always know more about the patient than the patient would know about the nurse. Like the first view, it acknowledges the depth or intensity of NPRs. Unlike friendship, one-sided intimacy fails to account for the personal and professional growth nurses experience by virtue of their daily witnessing of human suffering. When trying to learn knowledge or skill, we often seek an analogy or metaphor that will help us understand or give us a framework (e.g., this will feel like a toothache or it is like riding a bicycle). The contrasting views of NPRs and the characterization of a patient's need for a nurse as a need for hand-holding highlight the poverty of language and a failure of cultural imagination. At some level, the culture in which we practice has recognized the intimacy of therapeutic relationships that nurses establish with patients, mostly expressed in degrading media caricatures of female nurses. Describing the interpersonal process nurses use to help patients use coaching enriches the clinical language and moral imagination clinicians bring to their encounters with sufferers.

I believe that the intimacy of the NPR deserves more exploration and explanation if the full potential of the profession in alleviating suffering is to be achieved. To characterize the NPR as friendship is dangerous. It denies the mutuality of friendship (e.g., expectations). It can set nurses up for unrealistic expectations of patients. For patients, the NPR as friendship could be nontherapeutic since, using this model, nurses might feel free to unburden themselves to patients and families. The question remains—how is a nurse (or any clinician) to process and understand intense emotions elicited in NPRs. In addition to the therapeutic issues, the friendship paradigm suggests that a clinical discipline which depends on interpersonal competence is simply a human skill. Therefore, anyone can do it so why should it be studied or funded? Furthermore, it denies the conscious use and interpretation of complex cognitive, affective, and behavioral knowledge acquired during professional education that enable clinicians to communicate deliberately for the purpose of effecting therapeutic goals.

The culture in which we practice offers no models for the deep emotions evoked by relationships with patients, especially if they exist over time as is the case when caring for those who are chronically ill or dying. Nurse-patient relationships can evoke the most tender and fiercest of emotions—love, sadness, and anger. The usual arenas for expressing such intense emotions are within families, or between confidantes or lovers. If these feelings are not identified and addressed in an atmosphere of comfort and safety during student learning experiences, then nurses and other clinicians are likely to flounder. They will misinterpret their emotional responses to clinical experiences and lose the ability to be therapeutic, becoming either "overinvolved" or detached and burnt out. It is important to understand the essence of encounters between nurses and patients and between nurses and patients' families, if we are to prepare compassionate clinicians who can humanize the environments in which illness and suffering are experienced.

Like love, pain, or birth, trying to find language to capture the privileges, emotions, and interactions inherent in profound encounters between nurses and patients is, as Donna Diers would say, like "nailing jello to the wall." The results of my quest for this language led me to coaching, first mentioned by Benner (12), as a word whose meaning would be educational, sustaining, and descriptive of therapeutic relationships. Coaching simultaneously captures the expertise the nurse brings to NPRs, its intimate character, the emotions evoked, and the possibilities for personal growth for both nurses and patients.

Suffering

The selective literature review includes theoretical and investigative work that address the intrapersonal, interpersonal, and social aspects of suffering. This approach is taken to provide a basis for examining coaching as the essence of the interpersonal process nurses use to guide and comfort those who suffer.

Conceptual Work on Suffering and Pain

Suffering is a whole person concept (3), (13), (14). Frank (15), a psychotherapist and concentration camp survivor, wrote that suffering is part of the human condition and that it is one of the ways humans find meaning in life. The role of the clinician is to "enlist the patient's capacity to fulfill the meaning of his suffering" (15, p. 188). He emphasized that suffering is unavoidable and can be ennobling. Suffering is one way humans are able to find meaning in life. Even when all freedoms appear to be lost, one exercises freedom by choosing one's attitude and searching for meaning. He maintained that humans can retain their dignity, even though they may lose their usefulness.

Cassell (13) defined suffering as the "state of severe distress associated with events that threaten the intactness of the person" (13, p. 640). "Suffering occurs when an impending destruction of the person is perceived; it continues until the threat of disintegration has passed or until the integrity of the person can be restored in some other manner" (14, p. 33). Reflecting on patients' experiences of illness and suffering, he described the many aspects of a person that can be sources of, or affected by, suffering: personality, character, the past, life experiences, family, cultural background, roles, relationships, the self, one's rights and responsibilities, the body, one's activities and regular behaviors, the unconscious, one's secret life, a perceived future, and transcendence (or a life of the spirit) (13), (14). These facts of a person assist in understanding the complexity of suffering but persons cannot be reduced to subjective knowing, mind, or spirituality (14). Suffering is often associated with pain but it can occur when any dimension of the person is threatened.

Copp described suffering as "the state of anguish of one who bears pain, injury, or loss" (16, p. 491). Copp (17) subsequently described nine concepts that make up the construct of suffering: vulnerability, dehumanization, self-concept, coping, mind-body concepts, time, place, stress, and meaning and purpose. There are six categories of vulnerability: potential, temporary, circumstantial, episodic, permanent and inevitable (17). The idea of vulnerability suggests that clinicians can identify those "at risk for" suffering. In a further exploration of suffering, Copp and Copp (18) described ways providers "dispirit" patients. Practices which intimidate or dispirit are treating patients as objects or as invisible; blaming patients for their pain or for not behaving cheerfully; failing to consult patients about their participation in care; and not listening to patients. Kahn and Steeves, expanding on existing definitions of suffering, described suffering as the experience of having "some crucial aspect of one's own self, being, or existence is threatened" (7, p. 626). An important contribution of these authors is the recognition that suffering is not necessarily a perception or sensation but an evaluation of the significance or meaning of experiences that can induce suffering (7), (19).

Two authors have explored the process of suffering. Drawing on religious and other literature, Soelle (20) described three phases of suffering. In the first phase, an individual is mute and speechless, overwhelmed by the situation, powerless, and submissive; autonomy is lost and goals cannot be organized. The second phase is lamentation—the sufferer finds a voice, suffering is experienced, accepted and analyzed; efforts are made to conquer suffering and goals are established. The third phase is characterized by action—objectives are organized, the individual attempts to shape the situation and overcome powerlessness. Battenfield (21) developed a conceptual schema of responses to suffering. She, too, described three phases. The initial impact is immobilizing. The second phase, turmoil without resolution, is characterized by many negative emotions such as guilt and anger. Recovery is characterized by effective coping, acceptance and finding meaning. This schema is a "progression" (21, p. 36). and can be criticized for its linearity. In chronic illness, the continuum is likely to be dynamic. People who suffer may never recover meaning, or they may find meaning but then lose their grasp of it when illness relapses or another crisis occurs. These dynamic aspects of suffering are echoed in a call for more ethnographic studies of suffering (22) and in grounded theory studies of chronic illness (23) which suggest that patients may be able to shape illness trajectories.

Research

Intrapersonal, interpersonal, and social dimensions of suffering: the patient's perspective.   The Quality of Life (QOL) tool used at City of Hope was developed from the perspective of cancer patients (24). Patients with chronic cancer pain were asked to identify attributes that defined the content domain of quality of life. Three broad categories of attributes of quality of life for patients with cancer related pain emerged—physical and psychological well-being and interpersonal concerns (24). Subsequent studies revealed that spiritual well-being was also an important aspect of QOL (25). The model, Impacts of Pain on the Dimensions of Quality of Life (25) (Figure 9–1, page 213) indicates that QOL as defined by patients with cancer pain is a multidimensional construct with intrapersonal and interpersonal dimensions. The intrapersonal dimensions include physical functioning and symptoms, affective states associated with the presence or absence of pain, and spiritual issues including suffering and the meaning of pain.

Based on her program of research, Kolcaba (26), (27) proposed that comfort be used as an holistic outcome measure. The bidimensional taxonomic structure of comfort is illustrated in Figure 8–1. One dimension is the intensity of comfort needs which represents a continuum—relief, ease, and transcendence. The second dimension consists of four subscales: physical, psychospiritual, environmental, and social. Interestingly, this model of comfort overlaps with Ferrell and colleagues' model of patient-defined QOL. As in the QOL model, there is a physical dimension that refers to the experience of bodily sensations. The psychospiritual dimension pertains to aspects of the self, meaning, and spirituality. The social dimension corresponds closely with the social concerns identified in the QOL model. Kolcaba added another dimension not identified in the QOL model, that of the environment, which addresses the contribution of one's immediate surroundings to comfort. As she has conceptualized comfort, it might be the opposite of suffering (rather than discomfort). Extending Kolcaba's analysis, comfort could be viewed as a vital and desirable clinical outcome of effective interventions for suffering. The sources of suffering would not have to be removed nor cured for the sufferer to feel better.

Kodiath and Kodiath's (28) grounded theory study of people with chronic noncancer pain from two different cultures revealed a basic psychological problem and a basic social psychologic process (Figure 8–2). Differences between Americans and Asian Indians emerged throughout the process. These differences were characterized on the basis of meaning. Chronic pain in Indians led to a quest for meaning, the outcomes of which were integration, spiritual surrender, and increased support from loved ones. Americans with chronic pain embarked on a quest for cure, the outcomes of which were disintegration, hopeless surrender, and separation or distance from loved ones. This is an important contribution to understanding the phenomenon of

FIGURE 8–1   *Taxonomic Structure of Comfort*

INTENSITY OF UNMET/MET COMFORT NEEDS

	Relief	Ease	Transcendence
Physical			
Psychospiritual			
Environmental			
Social			

DEGREE OF INTERNAL/EXTERNAL NEEDS

DIMENSION ONE

Relief— the experience of a patient who has a specific need met.

Ease — a state of calm or contentment.

Transcendence — the state in which one rises above problems or pain.

DIMENSION TWO

Physical— pertaining to bodily sensations.

Psychospiritual— pertaining to the internal awareness of self, including esteem, concept, sexuality and meaning in one's life; can also encompass one's relationship to a higher order or being.

Environmental— pertaining to the external background of human experience; encompasses light, noise, ambience, color, temperature, and natural versus synthetic elements.

Social— pertaining to interpersonal, family, and societal relationships.

Source: Reprinted with permission from Kolcaba, K. (1991). A taxonomic structure for the concept of comfort. Image, 23, 235–238.

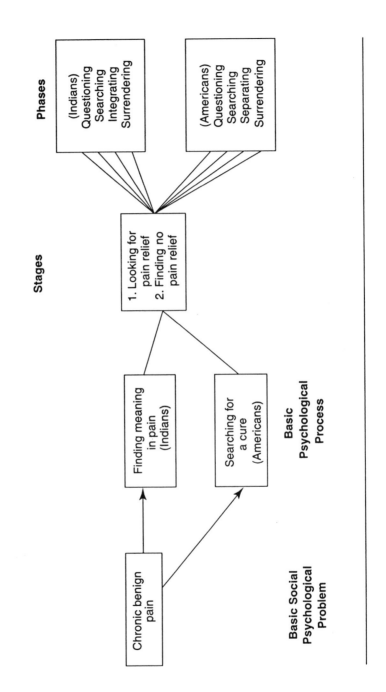

FIGURE 8-2 The Substantive Theory—Major Theoretical Constructs

Phases

(Indians)
Questioning
Searching
Integrating
Surrendering

(Americans)
Questioning
Searching
Separating
Surrendering

Stages

1. Looking for pain relief
2. Finding no pain relief

Finding meaning in pain (Indians)

Searching for a cure (Americans)

Basic Psychological Process

Chronic benign pain

Basic Social Psychological Problem

183

chronic pain and the potential influence of culture on pain and suffering. Because finding meaning emerged as a central aspect of the theory and seemed to explain differences between the two groups, it is relevant to suffering.

Using a qualitative approach, Benedict (29) sought to determine the incidence of suffering associated with the experience of lung cancer. A structured interview elicited whether subjects had experienced a list of physical, psychological, and interactional factors that had been identified in a previous investigation of suffering. Disability was the most frequently reported cause of suffering. Fifty per cent of the sample indicated that they experienced very much or a lot of suffering related to disability. Pain was the second most common factor associated with suffering; 40 percent reported very much or a lot of suffering. Subjects with known metastases were compared with those who had no known metastases. There was a statistically significant difference between those with metastases and those without in the amount of suffering due to psychological causes. There were no significant differences on physical or interactional cause of suffering between the two groups. Although suffering is an individual experience, this study suggests that common sources of suffering can be identified in a group of patients with the same diagnosis. The most common ones, disability and pain, are amenable to nursing interventions.

Some studies illustrate the interpersonal dimension of suffering from the perspective of the patient. Charmaz (30) studied how suffering undermines the self and identified psychological conditions that contribute to suffering. Seventy-three in-depth interviews with 57 chronically ill individuals were analyzed. Four themes related to the self and suffering were identified: living a restricted life, social isolation, discrediting definitions of self (stigma), and becoming a burden. The notion of stigma as an aspect of suffering is particularly interesting since it is most often a social process in which the sufferer is "labeled" by others who are well or not disabled. In a study of patients with chronic pain, perceived stigma was associated with pejorative clinician labeling, leading the investigators to urge clinicians to make efforts to reduce patients' feelings of estrangement. (31) The findings from these two studies suggest that interpersonal, communicative, and social dimensions of providing care are central to being therapeutic.

Cameron (32) generated a theory of Integrative Balancing (Table 8–1) that described the nature of comfort to a hospitalized patient as an active social process that has intrapersonal and interpersonal di-

TABLE 8–1   Integrative Balancing: The Basic Social Process

Stages	Phases	Characterized by:
1. Monitoring	• Watching • Interpreting • Measuring • Reducing	• Hyperalertness • Increased sensitivity • Protective hypervigilance
2. Networking	• Linking • Bonding • Acting • Supporting • Balancing	• Action and communication sets • Reciprocity, humour • "Acting to alter"
3. Enduring	• Waiting • Suffering • Hoping • Integrating	• Ambiguity • Reviewing the past • Revising • Regaining control

mensions. The patients' descriptions of comfort suggested that there is a continuum of comfort (Figure 8–3)—that "begins with a basic social problem causing discomfort and ends with achievement of high-level comfort" (p. 426). Integrative balancing consists of monitoring, networking, and enduring behaviors used by patients to alleviate discomfort and achieve comfort (Table 8–1). The stages of enduring are associated with suffering, waiting, and hoping and is characterized by ambiguity, reviewing the past, revising, and regaining control. The author concluded that while patients tended to initiate efforts to promote comfort during hospitalization, nurses could help patients identify and mobilize resources to facilitate this process.

FIGURE 8–3   The Comfort Continuum

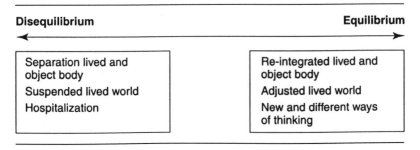

Intrapersonal, interpersonal and social aspects of suffering: caregiver perspectives.   The review thus far addresses suffering from the perspective of the patient. While the review of the conceptual work on suffering did not allude to a "community of sufferers," the snapshots of suffering suggest that suffering in one person elicits suffering in another. Families and professional caregivers often keep a vigil with the person who is dying or suffering from pain, illness, or other losses. How does witnessing suffering—keeping a vigil—affect loved ones and caregivers? The following evidence suggests that a "circle of suffering" may emerge from the suffering of one individual. It is likely that this secondary suffering depends on the nature, connection, and importance of the persons and relationships.

Interpersonal and social dimensions of quality of life led Ferrell and colleagues (25) to explore the impact of cancer pain on family caregivers. Interviews were conducted with family caregivers whose loved ones were being cared for in hospice, a community hospital, or a comprehensive cancer center. The study questions were: What are family members' descriptions of pain? What impact does pain have on caregivers? What are the primary questions and concerns expressed by caregivers regarding pain management? and What could nurses and physicians do to better manage pain? From content analysis of the data, four themes emerged regarding pain: anatomic description, hidden pain (the patient trying to hide pain from loved ones—unsuccessfully), family fear and suffering, and overwhelming and unendurable pain. Three themes related to family members' suffering are: helplessness, coping by denying feelings, and wishing for the loved one's death. Suffering-related themes regarding questions and concerns focused on: the future, understanding why, death, and fear about what to do at home. Family members said that providers could help by: being there/offering hope; explaining; being honest and listening; (addressing) addiction concerns; and giving medication. When caring for cancer patients, Ferrell urges nurses to assess suffering in family members since they experience distress directly related to the loved one's pain.

Secondary, hermeneutic narrative analyses from a perspective of suffering were done on interviews that had been conducted with bereaved mothers whose sons had died of AIDS (33). The purpose of the study was to gain an understanding of the suffering the mothers had experienced. Brief characterizations of the narratives are as follows: limiting the expression of love over a lifetime; a vigil of suffering; and leaving a dying son; and struggling with homosexuality. These narratives are discussed from a cultural anthropological perspective leading the authors to conclude that suffering is a universal human phenomenon shaped by macro- and micro-forces. Suffering also creates chaos, leading sufferers to "strive to maintain coherence, integrity and harmony in their lives" (33, p. 355).

Suffering in nursing home residents was explored by Starck using a qualitative field approach (34). To determine the extent to which management of suffering is a feature of the nursing home as an organization, Starck's study focused on two questions: What are the types of resident responses to suffering as perceived by nursing home staff? and How do nursing home staff manage residents who suffer? An inventory of 22 losses in four categories—physiologic, psychosocial, economic, and human spirit—were identified. Resident responses to suffering were perceived by staff to fall into one of three categories: overt complainer, covert complainer, and quiet sufferers; behaviors characterizing these responses were also identified.

Data analysis to address the second question in Starck's (34) study yielded a typology of staff responses to residents' suffering, which varied depending on whether the resident was a complainer or quiet. Quiet sufferers tended to get the most humane and positive responses from staff—affection, gifts, protection from unpleasant truths, and assumption of an extended family role. Overt complainers were placated, cajoled, or ignored by staff. Covert complainers were sanctioned for certain behaviors and families were counseled not to feel guilty. The results of this study are disturbing. While the suffering of the residents could be documented, the interventions of licensed vocational nurses (LVNs) (no RN direct caregivers were mentioned) seemed superficial and unfocused. There appeared to be no reflective or systematic effort to help residents cope with the suffering readily identified by helping them look for meaning, to redefine quality of life, or to otherwise comfort them. Rather, caregivers adopted discriminatory patterns of interaction with residents based on residents' behavioral responses to the losses and suffering experienced. While little can be made of one small study, these findings suggest that interpersonal competence and understanding of individual coping styles are important to humane, therapeutic interactions that effectively comfort those who suffer.

An investigation of what the hospice experience was like for family survivors and nurse caregivers (35) provided some insight into the characteristics of the social process of professional caregiving to one population of sufferers. Five broad themes emerged that were described from both family and nurse perspectives: nurses' ways of being, ways of doing, ways of knowing, ways of receiving and giving, and ways of welcoming a stranger. Families and nurses noted the importance of the nurse's knowledge of the dying process and the transcendent (a spiritual quality—the ability to get beyond and outside oneself to perceive, respond to, and be with the sufferer (4)). Nurses consistently spoke of the privilege of being entrusted with the care of the families' loved ones and being invited to share in the "intimate" experience of dying. Both nurses and families recognized the personal growth that resulted from the relationships established. Nurses spoke explicitly about their role in relieving suffering. Stiles (39) found that families of hospice patients were able to identify behaviors of nurses that were comforting: being available, listening, offering hope, sitting with, holding a hand, talking with, truth-telling, answering questions, and humor. Families in this study also described nurses' knowledge of the dying process and of transcendence as being essential. Stiles characterized the nurse's relationship to hospice families as "the Shining Stranger" (35). This brief summary of findings does not do justice to the richness and eloquence of the data and the depth of the shared experience of professional caregiving from the perspectives of nurses and families.

Common themes emerge from this selective literature review on suffering. The notion of self, the whole person, is central to understanding suffering. Persons may be suffering or be at risk for suffering, that is, vulnerable. Suffering is often associated with pain, hopelessness, powerlessness, or other physical and affective states. Suffering has temporal and intrapersonal dimensions. It is influenced by concerns from the past, and about the present and future. If often prompts a quest for meaning. Suffering can consume the individual, overwhelming one's intrapersonal resources and eliminating the simplest of pleasures. Both Soelle and Scarry (36) suggest that sufferers lose their voices figuratively or literally (e.g. the intubated patient).

Suffering is also a social process. It affects roles and relationships. The suffering of individuals can generate suffering in their loved ones and exhaust sources of social support. Involvement with suffering also influences professional caregiving, leading nurses to comfort and sustain or to diminish and abandon the sufferer. The challenge to sufferers and their caregivers is to find meaning, to transcend their situations, to recover from, or integrate, the experience. Nurses are also challenged to find meaning, cope with vulnerability, resist burnout, and learn how to comfort and sustain the patient. Kleinman (22, p. 129) in advocating the use of ethnography as a method for studying illness and suffering, asserted that ". . . suffering needs to be described and interpreted as part of the lived flow of *interpersonal* [emphasis added] experience in local moral worlds." The next sections explore the nurse-patient relationship as the central therapeutic intervention for comforting those who suffer.

Coaching: The Central Interpersonal Process in the Nurse-Patient Relationship (NPR)

Theoretical Work in Nursing

The relationships nurses establish with patients are crucial therapeutic interventions. The nurse must be skilled at establishing relationships that can be therapeutic regardless of the duration of the relationship. For many years, nurse researchers seemed to have abandoned the directions for research suggested by early conceptualizations of the NPR. This early work is compelling even today. Peplau conceptualized the NPR as a continuum (37). At the initial encounter the nurse and client have entirely separate goals and interests. They possess their own preconceptions of the meaning of the situation and the roles of each in the encounter. The initial encounter between nurse and patient is that of strangers; it is important to accept the person as she is *and* to treat the person as an emotionally able stranger. As they work together, they begin to have partial, mutual, and individual understandings of the nature of the situation, the roles of patient and nurse, and the requirements of each role. Through this process they arrive at a mutual understanding of the situation and establish common goals that focus on the patient. Ultimately, they engage in collaborative efforts directed toward solving or addressing the patients' health concerns. Nurses work with others to organize conditions that promote forward movement in health, personality, and other human processes in the direction of creative, constructive, productive, personal, and community living. Peplau recently characterized interpersonal relationships as ". . . the bedrock of quality of life" (p. 13). Sincere and trusting relationships with family members and good friends enable one to experience belonging, a sense of well-being, and social support; they also enhance one's ability to manage stress. Professional relationships and interactions are purposeful; they are resources to patients experiencing crises or making transitions which are aimed at producing outcomes beneficial for patients, such as enhanced coping.

According to Travelbee, the NPR is purposefully established and maintained by the nurse through the therapeutic use of self. She defined nursing as:

> an interpersonal process whereby the professional nurse practitioner assists an individual, family or community to prevent or cope with the experience of illness and suffering, and, if necessary, to find meaning in these experiences (the latter must not be evaded) (4).

She described the commitment involved in the relationship:

> It (the NPR) is to expose oneself to the shocks of commitment and all that this entails. It is to care and in the caring to be vulnerable but it is the vulnerability of the strong who are not afraid to be authentic human beings. It is the ability to face and confront reality—to face reality not as we wish it to be, but as it actually exists. Nurses must possess this trait if they would help others cope with the reality of illness and suffering. No one can give to others that which [she] does not [herself] possess. If nurses find no meaning in suffering, how can they assist others to face the reality of it, to cope with it, to bear and to somehow extract meaning or good out of such tragic experiences (4).

Possible outcomes of nurses' encounters with the crisis of personal vulnerability are detachment or transcendence. Only transcendence, the ability to get beyond and outside oneself to perceive, respond to, and be with the sufferer, enables nurses to be effective and grow—to focus on and help another while fully realizing one's own being. This caring "vitalizes and realizes the self; it does not annihilate it (4, p. 40).

Martocchio (8) described four characteristics of the NPR: authenticity, emotional closeness, self-representation, and belonging. *Authenticity* means being true to oneself—accepting responsibility for one's choices and being willing to make choices directed by one's values, personal identity, and life goals. *Emotional closeness* is a bonding characterized by openness to others and based on trust, not ownership or exclusiveness. It is a dance in which an atmosphere for closeness, not friendship, is created based on shared truths, shared feelings and self-knowledge. Emotional levels are high in such situations and nurses must accept these emotions; ignoring them subverts the possibilities for personal growth. Being open to sharing a common situation, being authentic, can contribute to a sense of belonging or feeling at home. *Belonging* enables us to represent ourselves honestly. This is vital if life is to have meaning, if individuals are to make choices that are authentic and consistent with their values. In an authentic NPR where an atmosphere of closeness and belonging have been created, nurses can protect patients from dehumanization and alienation and promote connection, meaning-making, growth, and development. Nurse and patient bring their whole selves—talents, needs, and wishes but the focus is on the patient's potentials and goals. "It is an intentional relationship, not an intimate friendship (8, p. 25). A key point that emerges from these three descriptions is that the NPR can be a source of education, personal growth, and self-actualization for patients and nurses.

Three nurses-authors suggest friendship as a model for the NPR. Rawnsley (9) is quite clear that the use of the term is metaphorical—it is *like* friendship, it is *not* friendship. It is also qualified with the word "instrumental"—suggesting that it is a tool or technique. Rawnsley (9) believes that instrumental friendship is a useful metaphor for understanding NPRs. Instrumental friendship is a means to some end as opposed to being an end in itself. Instrumental friendship changes as needs and goals change. In response to the distance and objectivity in NPRs that she had been taught, Polusny (10) proposes friendship as a paradigm for understanding and being effective in NPRs. The characteristics of friendship are discovery, learning, sharing, meeting, engaging, and connecting. Horner (11) describes the NPR as "intersubjective copresence." Intersubjectivity refers to the ability to apprehend the other's subjective world; realities are shared. One is willing to subjectively experience another's emotions as the basis for understanding. Copresence means each person involved in the encounter is fully present and aware of the other as a thinking, responding being. One brings one's whole self—body, emotions, and cognitions—to the situation and is aware of the other as a presence not an object. Intersubjective means "being receptive to the humanity in the other, so that an empathic encounter occurs" (p. 109). Both individuals, she maintains, are aware of sharing a unique experience.

One could probably characterize all human relationships as involving intersubjective copresence. Therapeutic NPRs depend on the ability of the nurse to apprehend the subjective world of the patient.

However, I would argue that as a professional nursing competency, establishing NPRs builds on a basic human trait. The nurse's personality, education, assessments, experiences, and intuition interact with affective, cognitive, and behavioral processes to enable the nurse to evaluate information from, and interactions with patients. Bonding or building a therapeutic relationship demands this deliberate, reflective approach to interpersonal interactions. Furthermore, though patients may wish to understand the subjective world of the nurse, suffering, illness, fatigue, and other factors compromise the stamina needed to arrive at such an understanding. To expect patients to try to be copresent in the way the nurse is is unrealistic for at least two reasons. It can divert the patient's limited physical and psychological energy from a focus on patient needs and goals and may undermine the therapeutic effectiveness of the NPR. The authors who use friendship as a model for understanding NPRs do not address mutuality, affection, and responsibility—characteristics of friendship, which if friendship is a viable paradigm, need to be discussed.

Theoretical Work on Coaching: An Interdisciplinary Perspective

This discussion is based on unpublished reviews of theoretical and investigative work on coaching from the fields of vocational rehabilitation, cognitive psychology, sport psychology, and music (38), (39). The emphasis in this section is on theoretical work. Research from these disciplines is used to inform the chapter's concluding synthesis and description of coaching.

Vocational rehabilitation (40).   Supported employment, also known as job coaching, refers to activities designed to help handicapped individuals obtain and sustain competitive employment. Job coaching encompasses three activities: assessment, intervention, and monitoring. A job coach thoroughly analyzes a prospective work environment. The coach then determines needs for job training and advocacy for the employee and initiates compensatory and adaptive strategies to ensure an acceptable standard of productivity. It is this activity that is the most time and labor intensive for the coach. Once competence has been demonstrated, the coach continues to monitor the employee's performance and adjustment.

Cognitive psychology.   Social skills tutoring (41) and Interpersonal Cognitive Problem Solving (ICPS) (42) are coaching techniques that have been used to help clients gain social skills and competence and improve their problem-solving abilities. Coaching may include features of contingency reinforcement and modeling but emphasizes specific instruction on target behaviors with opportunities to practice them and to receive feedback (43). Examples of target behaviors are: specific social skills (e.g., eye contact), language skills, and physical or motor skills. Both social skills tutoring and ICPS include direct verbal instructions in problem solving principles. ICPS also emphasizes thinking processes such as problem identification, generating alternative solutions, anticipating consequences of solutions, and cognitive context (43).

Sport psychology. Relationships among and between coaches and athletes are the basis of team functioning and the sources of motivation (44). Participation in sport is thought to affect many aspects of human development (45). Coach expectations can influence athlete performance (46) and self-esteem (47). Coaches are expected to have technical competence, interpersonal skills, communicating and motivating skills, and teaching, leadership and management skills (45), (48), (49). The absence of information about "player leadership" and descriptions of the "depth of mutual respect and caring that can develop between players and coaches" has been noted (50).

Using Rogerian humanism as a theoretical foundation, Lombardo described the humanistic coach. Humanism emphasizes holism, attention to subjective experience and feelings, challenge, psychological flexibility, creativity, imagination, and problem solving (45). The coach must be secure in his/her own self-concept, be self-accepting, and feel competent in order to be able to focus on the process of strengthening the athlete's self-concept. Humanistic coaches value athletes and communicate that athletes' goals, feelings, and opinions count. A coach conveys to athletes that they are trustworthy, responsible, capable of self-direction, and able to identify relevant goals. The coach is willing to discuss athletes' subjective experiences, address feelings, analyze behavior, and discuss personal meanings of their experiences.

Participation in sport contributes to the athlete's personal development (45). The coach creates and presents complex, difficult challenges to provide opportunities to discover performance abilities and develop the player's capacities. *Physical* development is enhanced. Players must focus on their bodies and learn strategies for achieving optimum performance. They learn how their bodies respond to the stress of athletic performance, fostering physical self-awareness and self-understanding. *Cognitive* development sharpens as individuals learn to

analyze, evaluate, and synthesize information from the coach, team-
mates, and self about performance and experience. Self-evaluation and
introspection are fostered. *Psychological* development is promoted. The
coach maximizes individual success by confirming and validating the
athlete, enabling the person to experience satisfaction, pride, self-esteem, enhanced self-concept, and self-confidence. Team sports refine
social skills through cooperation, interaction, and communication.
Sport also influences the affective domain, enabling the person to
experience enjoyment, disappointment, and a wide range of feelings
arising from interactions with teams, opponents, and coaches.

   Musical performance.   Acknowledging the elusiveness of the
meaning of art, Adler tried to convey the art of coaching and the depth
of human connection needed between coach and singer (51). Rather than
paraphrase, I quote directly from the text, substituting words relevant
to health care such as nurse and patient for coach, singer, and other
musical terms.

> The specific art of . . . coaching lies in the ability to deeply feel
> the [patient's] intentions and her artistry [talents and goals]; to
> attune oneself to [her . . . style of being and becoming]; to recognize
> [the patient's] shortcomings [needs] and to make up for them by
> extending a helping hand to lead [her], giving her a sense of . . .
> mastery and matching it by following [her] . . . coaching is a
> continuous give and take, a molding of two personalities into one
> . . . a coach must try to search for and understand where the roots
> of [the patient's individuality and being] lie . . . Faith—religious,
> metaphorical, or materialistic—is one of the strongest roots; faith
> in oneself is part of it; another root is [the ability to compensate]
> for shortcomings in one's makeup . . . [another is] sensitivity . . .
> Without sensitivity—the ability to feel influences from without
> and within and to [transform them] there can be no [becoming]
> (51, p. 82).

Research Relevant to the Nurse-Patient Relationship

In a recent study of patients, nurses, and chaplains relationships and
transcendence emerged as important categories for spiritual assessment
and intervention (52). Studies summarized in this section affirm the
intimate nature and therapeutic power of nurse-patient relationships
suggested by Travelbee (4), Martocchio (8), Peplau (37), and Stiles (35),
and would support the concept of coaching as a more accurate descrip-
tor of the NPR.

   Benner's qualitative research of nurses' clinical experiences identified seven domains of nursing practice (12). One domain was the

teaching-coaching role of the nurse. Competencies within this domain are listed in Table 8–2. Benner elaborated on the coaching role of clinical specialists (53). "Coaches learn what the illness means to the individual, what the adaptive demands, tasks and resources are for the patient at different stages in the illness" (53, p. 43). The expert coach has four main tasks: interpreting unfamiliar diagnostic and treatment demands; coaching the patient through alienated stances (e.g. anger, hopelessness, suffering); identifying changing relevance as demands or symptoms of the illness change; and ensuring cure is enhanced by care.

Coaching cannot be taught by precept—it requires a combination of experience and education (53). This combination of formal education and experience builds the nurse's repertoire of coaching interventions for particular situations. Benner defined experience from a phenomenological perspective as "the turning around, the adding of nuance, the amending or changing of preconceived notions or perceptions of the situation" (54, p. 21). "Practical knowledge resides in lived everyday understandings, meanings embodied in skillful comportment" (54, p. 3). Although she does not relate this to her prior work on coaching, her discussion of practical knowledge is relevant to developing one's coaching skills. In addition to demonstrating the teaching-coaching competencies identified by Benner, clinical specialists coach patients by making new developmental experiences approachable and understandable (55). Thus, becoming an effective coach depends on a combination of formal education and clinical experience. Over the course of caring for patients, nurses learn and understand the many ways people experience and cope with illness, pain, suffering, birth, and

---

TABLE 8–2   The Teaching-Coaching Role of the Nurse

· Timing–Capturing a patient's readiness to learn

· Assisting patients to integrate the implications of illness and recovery into their lifestyles

· Eliciting and understanding a patient's interpretation of his or her illness

· Providing an interpretation of the patient's condition and a rationale for procedures

· The coaching function: Making culturally avoided aspects of an illness approachable and understandable

Source: Benner, P. (1985). From novice to expert: Excellence and power in clinical practice. Menlo Park: Addison-Wesley Publishing Copany.

death. They use these experiences to help patients identify alternatives that enable them to understand, control, accept or triumph in the midst of unfamiliar experiences (12).

Using a Delphi approach, a nationwide survey of nurses was done to identify common nursing interventions (56). The purpose of the survey was to develop a classification of nursing interventions. One of the interventions was "Complex Relationship Building" defined as "Establishing a therapeutic relationship with a patient who has difficulty interacting with others" (58). This definition and the background references suggest that the intervention came from psychiatric nursing practice. However, many of the activities associated with the intervention characterize therapeutic relationships experienced by this author in her work with patients with cancer or chronic pain. An alternative definition of complex relationship building might be "establishing a therapeutic relationship with a patient whose nursing care needs require expert interpersonal knowledge and skill to achieve mutually determined outcomes." Examples might include patients with chronic physical or mental illness, patients and loved ones who are suffering, patients with chronic pain, or patients who are self-neglectful resulting in frequent utilization of emergency or episodic health care.

Lamb and Stempel were interested in learning what the experience of having nurse case managers was like for patients (57). Referral to nursing case management had occurred during a hospitalization for an acute event. Nurse Case Managers (NCMs) had been following the subjects for periods of time ranging from two months to two years. NCMs were not setting-bound; the duration and intensity of their interventions with patients were mutually determined. The grounded theory method was used to analyze interviews with 16 subjects. The basic social process (Figure 8–4) that emerged was that of individuals becoming their own insider-experts. During the stage of bonding, patients came to believe that the nurse knew how to help them and that patients felt "known" as persons. Patients identified activities of the nurses which seemed to facilitate a patient's development as insider: listening, validating, joking, touching, counseling, reframing, supporting, confronting, offering options, and praising. This stage seems to be a prerequisite to the stage of working when patients began to think differently about their illnesses. Nurses' demonstrated concern for patients appeared to be critical in bringing about cognitive changes that enabled them to explore attitudes and behaviors that tended to exacerbate illness and increase health care utilization. Thus, the first two stages are characterized by affective and cognitive changes in patients which they attribute to the case manager's care. The third stage, changing, described patients' implementation of behavioral changes. Two major behavioral changes reported were doing more for oneself and accepting help when needed. The authors concluded that for patients to grow as insider-experts and successfully manage the demands of chronic illnesses depended on the establishment of a strong interpersonal relationship between NCM and patient. This relationship enhances motivation and helps patients feel safe as they try out new behaviors. Observed outcomes included improved self-care, fewer hospitalizations, and improved quality of life.

Taken together, the literature on coaching and the NPR indicates that therapeutic relationships are complex processes with the potential to shape patients' experiences of illness and suffering. This review provided descriptions of coaching from other disciplines that are comparable to the coaching done by nurses in their interactions with patients. Clearly, coaching is more than hand-holding, though hand-holding, a type of comforting touch, is an important coaching activity. Coaching captures the essence of the relationship nurses create with patients upon which their effectiveness depends. It is a concept that has common meanings across disciplines and human experiences. It is a term that permits the experience of intense emotions on both sides; it captures the temporal nature of the relationship (which may be brief or extended); it suggests both the one-sided aspect (the coach has

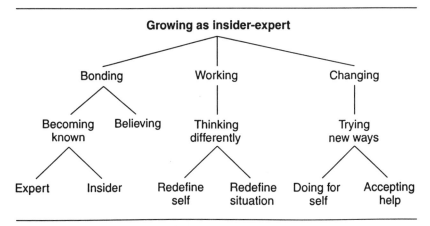

FIGURE 8–4   Growing as Insider-Expert

information and expertise needed by the patient) and the mutuality (opportunities for personal growth) in the relationship; and it conveys the contractural or voluntary nature of the relationship (if the relationship is not working despite the best efforts of both, another coach may need to be found).

Coaching Patients and Families Who Suffer

Analysis and synthesis of the literature reviewed here reveals dimensions of the person that affect or are affected by suffering, the processes nurses use to develop therapeutic relationships and ameliorate suffering, and possible patient outcomes. Persons cannot be reduced to aspects of their suffering and nurses must care for sufferers in a holistic manner. However, for instructional purposes, Table 8–3 summarizes the dimensions, processes, and outcomes extracted from the literature. Development of the table was also informed by work done by Miller (58) and Daloz (59). Table 8–3 illustrates the complexity of coaching as a therapeutic intervention. Readers should remember that patients can experience multiple sources of suffering simultaneously. Coaching is a dynamic process, so that several behaviors may be used at once. Patient outcomes may occur at the moment of interaction or emerge over time. Recognizing the dimensions of personhood most affected by suffering enables nurses to channel their communications and behaviors in ways that are most likely to be effective. The list of coaching behaviors can be used by nurses and other clinicians to evaluate their therapeutic relationships and activities they use to provide comfort and ameliorate suffering.

TABLE 8–3   Coaching Behaviors: Interventions to Comfort Sufferers

Dominant Dimension of Personhood Affected by Suffering	**Coaching Behavior**	**Possible Outcomes**
Bodily (physical)	• Positioning • Pain & symptom management • Providing hygiene, toileting, & other physical interventions while preserving dignity	• Self- or caregiver report of improved physical comfort • Improved function

Affective, Psychological, and/or Spiritual	• Accepting person as he/she is • Acknowledging person's courage & strength • Being available/present • Being honest/telling the truth • Bonding • Comforting by touch & words • Counseling • Eliciting meaning patient ascribes to situation • Eliciting patient and caregiver expectations, fears • Encouraging, praising • Ensuring safe passage • Inspiring/inspiriting • Listening • Keeping a vigil • Offering hope • Reassuring • Supporting • Validating	• elf-acceptance • Improved self-worth • Self-report of transcendence and/or new meaning • Revised future agendas • Improved quality of life • Decreased anxiety • Hope • Accepts help from others • Increased ability to initiate self-care • Self-report of satisfaction with decision-making
Cognitive/ Behavioral	• Challenging • Confronting/identifying contradictions • Demonstrating • Discussing • Explaining • Guiding • Modeling • Monitoring • Motivating • Offering a map • Offering options • Organizing goals • Providing feedback • Reframing expectations, goals, meanings • Setting tasks • Teaching • Using humor	• Behavior change • Self-report of fining meaning, new attitudes, more coping strategies • Identifies and uses cognitive coping strategies • Uses self-care behaviors to increase comfort, & decrease suffering
Social	• Advocating • Bonding • Collaborating with patient, family, other providers • Communicating • Facilitating important relationships • Keeping tradition	• Affection • Asks for help • Comfort • Social support • Patient satisfaction with care

Dimensions of Personhood Affected by Suffering: Assessment

The initial encounter between nurse and patient usually sets the tone for future interactions. Nurses must attend to creating a trusting partnership and a context that will enable them to help the sufferer. It is important to believe the patient and make a commitment to help. Nurses often cannot promise patients and families that suffering will disappear; however, they *can* reassure patients that they will not be abandoned.

Assessment can identify those who are vulnerable or at risk for suffering. Patient reports of prior negative experiences with health care can be used by the nurse to initiate preventive interventions. For example, a colleague had gynecological surgery associated with an extremely difficult postoperative course, largely due to inadequate pain management and consequent suffering. Two years later, when further surgery was needed, she enlisted her physician and primary nurse to help her plan a different, more positive experience. This planning was so successful, she characterized the experience as a "designer hospitalization." Although pain could not be eliminated, environmental and other factors were able to be modified to ensure a more positive experience.

Suffering often has multiple antecedents, so assessment of the person suffering is vital to identify factors that can be eliminated or modified and those that may be amenable to exploration of alternative meanings or coping strategies. Antecedents include those that are physical, psychological (including cognitive and affective aspects), spiritual, and environmental (3). From the assessment, factors that cause or exacerbate suffering are identified—for example, pain, disability, unfinished business, fractured relationships, or despair. Assessment should also reveal personal qualities, environmental, and social factors that ameliorate suffering—for example, courage, values, spiritual resources, past experience with similar situations, familiar objects (e.g., a pillow), and social support. During assessment, nurses should be mindful of the community of sufferers within the patient's social circle. Nurses assess social factors that influence suffering, including the patient's relationship with family members, health care professionals, and others to identify interpersonal interactions that undermine the patient's ability to cope with or transcend suffering. Intervening with a significant other or collaborating with another provider can comfort the patient or a patient's loved one. A more complete discussion of assessment of sources of suffering is available (3). As with any clinical concern, ongoing assessment and monitoring reveals interventions that are working and those that need to be modified.

Coaching Behaviors: Intervention

From the quote that opens the chapter, one is compelled to ask "Why were Mesdames Parent and Martin able to comfort de Beauvoir's mother when Madame Gontrand, who appeared to be doing the exact same things, could not?" I believe the answer lies in the interpersonal qualities of the nurses. Coaching can be considered an interpersonal intervention that requires the therapeutic use of self—one's mind, past experience, words, heart, and hands—to comfort those who suffer. The nurse relates to patients and families in ways that facilitate expression of feelings, help them find meaning, and redefine quality of life (3). The nurse as coach brings to relationshps with patients her whole self including commitments, understandings, vulnerability, personal knowing, authenticity, experiences, formal education, interpersonal and technical competence, and personality (3), (4), (8), (53), (60). A deliberate and reflective approach to the therapeutic relationship, one that attends to the unique concerns of the sufferer, is essential. Nurses use self-knowledge, personality, active listening skills, perspective-taking, and deliberative communications to understand experiences of suffering. The therapeutic relationship enables the nurse to understand the patient. This understanding can be used to increase the sensitivity of family members and health professionals to the imposed powerlessness experienced by patients (57).

While other disciplines provide psychological, spiritual, cognitive, and social interventions, the provision of physical or bodily comfort is largely in the realm of nurses. Pain and disability, factors associated with suffering, can lead to losses that make the sufferer dependent on others for the most basic and private of human functions. Assisting people with toileting and hygiene functions may appear menial to the non-nurse. In fact, needing assistance with these functions is often a source of profound embarrassment, if not suffering. Coaching that preserves human dignity and acknowledges the significance of loss of physical functions is integrated into these apparently mundane interventions.

Nurses address physical comfort in other ways—for example, pain, symptom, and illness management. The work by Stiles (35) and

Lamb and Stempel (57) suggest that to help patients to manage their illnesses, nurses get to know them the way sport coaches get to know an athlete's capabilities and limitations. Nurses need to teach patients and family members new skills or ways to modify previously acquired skills or habits—how to take medications; how to manage venous access devices, ostomies, and other treatments; positions that minimize pain; or more efficient ways of breathing.

Nurses also help patients develop and sustain psychological resources such as self-esteem, assertiveness, competence, and social support to enhance coping. I have found that being explicit in acknowledging patients' strengths and pointing out contradictions is a particularly useful coaching activity. These are examples of what Miller calls this "reality surveillance" (58). Patients sometimes get lost in the "swamp" of their illnesses—managing family and work so they can get to appointments; dealing with the recurrent assaults of an illness or a prolonged hospitalization; or coping with the demands of treatment (this blood test, those drugs). They lose sight of the strengths that enable them to cope with multiple physical and psychological demands. Acknowledging their courage and finding out "what keeps them going" can help them reframe their situations and recover a sense of self.

For example, a patient newly admitted to a rehabiliation hospital reported that she was overwhelmed but had difficulty identifying a particular aspect that was eliciting these findings. In the course of talking to her, her primary nurse pointed out that for the last seven years she had received care for her cancer at an acute care hospital, and that part of what was hard was dealing with a whole new staff and not being seen by the providers she had seen for seven years. She also asked the patient whether this was the first time she had been discharged to another hospital rather than home. To help the patient gain the rehabilitation staff's trust, the nurse and physician spoke with the patient's oncology physician or nurse practitioner daily, reporting on the patient's progress. These conversations were reported to the patient who was reassured that collaboration and communication were occurring on her behalf. The two alternative meanings offered by the nurse helped the patient see why this hospitalization felt SO different from her prior experiences. At a certain point, the patient was able to say, "I see why my oncologist wanted me here. Had I gone home I would have been incapable of doing things I would need to do and would have expected myself to be able to do."

Another intervention, commonly used by nurses when working

with the chronically ill, is "offering a map" (58) or anticipatory guidance. The nurse uses past experiences to prepare patients for what might lie ahead. Textbooks and research articles tend to describe what happens to groups of patients who have a particular diagnosis or get a particular treatment. Education, experience, pattern recognition, and intuition enable the nurse to tailor the map to the individual. The nurse synthesizes an understanding of biology, pharmacology, and other sciences with observations of real experiences with real patients to individualize coaching. One can compare this kind of coaching to that which occurs in music or ice skating. I believe professional nurses are unique among health care providers in having both a grasp of biological sciences and sustained contact with patients (measured in hours in institutional care or number of visits in home and hospice care). These characteristics enable them to provide a map that anticipates suffering (and other experiences), offers preventive or coping strategies, and projects possible destinations (outcomes).

Coaching Through Suffering: Outcomes

Both the theoretical and investigative work reviewed on suffering and the NPR suggest that physical and psychological comfort may be an outcome of nurses' interpersonal and educational interventions. The importance of finding meaning in pain and suffering, and patients' and families' efforts to do so have been described (3), (4), (6), (7), (17), (25), (28), (60). This implies that eliciting meanings patients ascribe to their suffering should be a priority for assessment. Possible outcomes of coaching behaviors to comfort sufferers are listed in Table 8–3. This list makes outcomes of caring for sufferers appear neater than they are in real life. Suffering and coaching are dynamic phenomena. Assessment should reveal desirable outcomes, ones that are consistent with the patient's values and definition of quality of life. Like the athletic coach, the nurse assesses the patient's existing capacities and potential for being comforted. For some sufferers, specific goals are realistic and attainable, even if the goal requires considerable effort. For others, alternative outcomes may need to be proposed. It may be a simple matter of revising expectations about timing or breaking expected outcomes into steps. For a patient suffering from pain, a revised outcome might be improving the quality and quantity of sleep, before expecting relief of pain. For other patients, learning ways to live or cope with uncertainty is an alternative to wanting definitive answers.

Patients and families carry in their heads numerous images and meanings that influence their expectations regarding suffering. Eliciting these images and offering accurate information can do much to comfort. One family member caring for a dying relative at home imagined that at the moment of death, the patient's body would explode. Many cancer patients remember a beloved friend or relative who died in agony. Reassuring them that nearly all cancer pain can be treated effectively can be a source of comfort.

Conclusion

Coaching as an interpersonal process captures the depth and importance of the nurse-patient relationship to effective comforting. The nurse/coach uses knowledge gained from education, experience, and patient assessment to provide patients with alternative interpretations regarding their experiences of health and illnesses. Through coaching, patients are offered a repertoire of possible behavioral, cognitive, and affective responses to unfamiliar situations and feelings. In this chapter, I have tried to describe a clinical skill—coaching as an interpersonal competence—that is sometimes recognized but rarely discussed in ways that demonstrate its complexity.

While suffering is a holistic phenomenon, ministering to sufferers usually takes place within contexts in which time, money, and productivity are valued. I have deliberately used the language of assessment and quality improvement (which can regarded as reductionistic) to help clinicians make visible the suffering of their patients and the complexity of comforting interventions that are low tech and interpersonal. It is interesting to note that in job coaching, an intervention to improve productivity of handicapped employees, the intervention phase was the most time and labor intensive for the coach (40).

The following scenario captures several aspects of coaching including: recognizing patient expectations, timing, vulnerability, deliberate use of words to convey alternative meanings, and seeing something the patient could not see from the "swamp" of his illness and pain.

> Mr. R. came to the clinic in severe pain. He was being followed by a hospice but they had not been successful in alleviating his pain. He was dejected, no eye contact, slumped in the chair (he's probably thinking if hospice wasn't able to help, how will you be

able to?). At the end of my assessment, I felt confident in assuring him that we were not "at the bottom of the bag of tricks." I thought he should be hospitalized so that we could try things quickly and monitor his responses. He did not want to be hospitalized (afraid he would never leave) so we made a plan for outpatient management. We had the same difficulty hospice did—therapeutic response to medications complicated by idiosyncratic responses and side effects that could not be corrected quickly enough and a man too tired and discouraged to try relaxation. After giving him a new "map" (with alternative possibilities), he agreed to hospitalization. However, in his effort to use a connection to facilitate hospital admission, he, in fact, lost the bed that had been available. He wanted to go home, his old fear of dying in the hospital reactivated by this glitch. I begged him to give me an hour to find another bed. I could not keep the tears of anguish and frustration from welling in my eyes. I believed his pain could be relieved and I believed that this was my LAST chance to help him—it would no longer matter how full my bag of tricks was if he lost his motivation to try. He waited. Four days later he was pain-free (on a combination of low-dose steroids, long-acting morphine, and relaxation), sitting up in bed, smiling and looking me in the eye. I sat with him. We ended up debriefing his experience with the pain team. He said, "That day in the clinic, when you told me we were not at the bottom of the bag of tricks, you gave me so much hope." Later, in talking about the hospitalization, he said, "I really wanted to go home. I was discouraged and mad. When I looked at you, you looked ready to cry. I couldn't believe you cared so much and I remembered what you said about the bag of tricks. I knew then that I should stay and wait while you did what you could to find a bed. And here I am; I feel good; I'm eating again; my wife and I will be able to take Pat (their developmentally disabled daughter) out for weekly dinners again, for a while anyway. I understand my pain better. The tapes (relaxation) help me sleep. I can't believe it. How can I thank you?"

This experience is a sustaining narrative (54), one that I retrieve when I am with a patient who suffers. Such narratives become part of nurses' repertoires for comforting, enabling us to face suffering again and again. For the reflective nurse, suffering is a teacher. Daily involvement with suffering and making and remaking meaning, demands that nurses examine their own lives, vaules, choices, and definitions of quality of life. As witnesses to the suffering of others, we are called upon to make sense of our own lives and experience personal growth so that we can continue to be present to those who need intelligent, compassionate comforting.

References

1. De Beauvoir, S. (1973). *A very easy death.* New York: Warner Paperback Library.
2. Alsop, S. 1973. *Stay of execution: A sort of memoir.* Philadelphia: J. B. Lippincott Company.
3. Spross, J. (1994). Pain, suffering, and spiritual well-being: Assessment and interventions. *Quality of life: A nursing challenge, 2,* 71–79.
4. Travelbee, J. (1971). *Interpersonal aspects of nursing.* Philadelphia: F. A. Davis Company.
5. Duffy, M. E. (1992). A theoretical and empirical review of the concept of suffering. In P. L. Starck & J. P. McGovern (Eds.), *The hidden dimension of illness: Human suffering* (pp. 291–303). New York: National League for Nursing Press.
6. Starck, P. L., & McGovern, J. P. (1992). The meaning of suffering. In P. L. Starck & J. P. McGovern (Eds.), *The hidden dimension of illness: Human suffering.* New York: National League for Nursing Press.
7. Kahn, D. L., & Steeves, R. H. (1986). The experience of suffering: Conceptual clarification and theoretical definition. *Journal of Advanced Nursing, 11,* 623–631.
8. Martocchio, B. (1987). Authenticity, belonging, emotional closeness, and self representation. *Oncology Nursing Forum, 14,* 23–27.
9. Rawnsley, M. (1990). Of human bonding: The context of nursing as caring. *Advances in Nursing Science, 13,* 41–48.
10. Poslusny, S. (1991). Friendship as paradigm for nursing science: Using scientific subjectivity and ethical interaction to promote understanding and social change. In R. M. Neil & R. Watts (Eds.), *Caring and nursing: Explorations in feminist perspectives* (pp. 163–172). New York: National League for Nursing.
11. Horner, S. (1991). Intersubjective copresence in a caring model. In R. M. Neil & R. Watts (Eds.), *Caring and nursing: Explorations in feminist perspectives* (pp. 107–116). New York: National League for Nursing.
12. Benner, P. (1984). *From novice to expert: Excellence and power in clinical practice.* Menlo Park: Addison-Wesley Publishing Company.
13. Cassell, E. (1982). The nature of suffering and the goals of medicine. *New England Journal of Medicine, 306,* 639–645.
14. Cassell, E. (1991). *The nature of suffering.* New York: Oxford University Press.
15. Frankl, V. (1963). *Man's search for meaning: An introduction to logotherapy.* New York: Pocket Books.
16. Copp, L. A. (1974). The spectrum of suffering. *American Journal of Nursing, 74,* 491–495.
17. Copp, L. (1990). The nature and prevention of suffering. *Journal of Professional Nursing, 6,* 247–249.
18. Copp, L. A., & Copp, J. D. (1993). Illness and the human spirit. *Quality of Life: A Nursing Challenge, 2,* 50–55.
19. Steeves, R., & Kahn, D. (1987). Experience of meaning in suffering. *Image: Journal of Nursing Scholarship, 19,* 114–116.
20. Soelle, D. (1975). *Suffering.* Philadelphia: Fortress Press.
21. Battenfield, B. L. (1984). Suffering—A conceptual description and context analysis of an operational schema. *Image: Journal of Nursing Scholarship, 16,* 36–41.

22. Kleinman, A. (1992). Local worlds of suffering: An interpersonal focus for ethnographies of illness experience. *Qualitative Health Research, 2,* 127–134.

23. Corbin, J. M. & Strauss, A. (1992). A nursing model for chronic illness management based upon the trajectory framework. In Woog, P. (Ed.), *The chronic illness trajectory framework: The Corbin and Strauss Nursing Model.* New York: Springer Publishing Co.

24. Padilla, G. V., Ferrell, B. R., Grant, M., et al. (1990). Defining the content domain of quality of life for cancer patients with pain. *Cancer Nursing, 13,* 108–115.

25. Ferrell, B. R., Rhiner, M., Zichi-Cohen, M., & Grant, M. (1991). Pain as metaphor for illness. Part I: Impact of cancer pain on family caregivers. *Oncology Nursing Forum, 18,* 1303–1309.

26. Kolcaba, K. (1991). A taxonomic structure for the concept comfort. *Image: Journal of Nursing Scholarship, 23,* 237–240.

27. Kolcaba, K. (1992). Holistic comfort: Operationalizing the construct as a nurse-sensitive outcome. *Advances in Nursing Science, 15,* 1–10.

28. Kodiath, M. F., & Kodiath, A. (1992). A comparative study of patients with chronic pain in India and the United States. *Clinical Nursing Research, 1,* 278–291.

29. Benedict, S. (1989). The suffering associated with lung cancer. *Cancer Nursing, 12,* 34–40.

30. Charmaz, K. (1983). Loss of self: A fundamental form of suffering in the chronically ill. *Sociology of Health and Illness, 5,* 168–195.

31. Marbach, J. J., Lennon, M. C., Link, B. G., & Dohrenwend, B. P. (1990). Losing face: Sources of stigma as perceived by chronic facial pain patients. *Journal of Behavioral Medicine, 13,* 583–604.

32. Cameron, B. (1993). The nature of comfort to hospitalized medical surgical patients. *Journal of Advanced Nursing, 18,* 424–436.

33. Gregory, D., & Longman, A. (1992). Mothers' suffering: Sons who died of AIDS. *Qualitative Health Research, 2,* 334–357.

34. Starck, P. (1992). The management of suffering in a nursing home: An ethnographic study. In P. Starck & J. McGovern (Eds.), *The hidden dimension of illness: Human suffering* (pp. 127–154). New York: National League for Nursing Press.

35. Stiles, M. (1990). The shining stranger: Nurse-family spiritual relationship. *Cancer Nursing, 13,* 235–245.

36. Scarry, E. (1985). *The body in pain: The making and unmaking of the world.* New York: Oxford University Press.

37. Peplau, H. E. (1952). *Interpersonal relations in nursing: A conceptual frame of reference.* New York: G. P. Putnam.

38. Spross, J. A. (1994). *State of the science: A review of interdisciplinary perspectives on coaching.* Unpublished manuscript, Boston College, Doctoral Program in Nursing, Chestnut Hill, MA.

39. Spross, J. A. (1994). *Chronic pain: A path to becoming.* Unpublished manuscript, Boston College, Chestnut Hill, MA.

40. Wehman, P., Kreutzer, J., West, M., Sherron, P. Zasler, N., Groah, C., Stonnington, H., Burns, C., & Sale, P. (1990). Return to work for persons with traumatic brain injury: A supported employment approach. *Archives of Physical Medicine and Rehabilitation, 71,* 1047–1052.

41. Frisch, M., Elliott, C., Atsaides, J., Salva, D., & Denney, D. (1982). Social skills and stress management training to enhance patients' interpersonal competencies. *Psychotherapy: Research and Practice, 19,* 349–358.

42. Hops, H. (1983). Children's social competence and skill: Current research practices and future directions. *Behavioral Therapy, 14,* 3–18.
43. Pelligrini, D., & Urbain, E. (1985). An evaluation of interpersonal cognitive problem solving training with children. *Journal of Psychology and Psychiatry, 26,* 17–41.
44. Sullivan, P., & Wilson, D. (1991). The coach's role. In G. Cohen (Ed.), *Women in sport: Issues and controversies* (pp. 230–237). Newbury Park: Sage Publications.
45. Lombardo, B. (1987). *The humanistic coach: From theory to practice.* Springfield, IL: Charles C. Thomas, Publisher.
46. Martinek, T., Crowe, P., & Rejeski, W. (1982). *Pygmalion in the gym: Causes and effects of expectations in teaching and coaching.* West Point, NY: Leisure Press.
47. Smith, R. & Smoll, F. (1991). Behavioral research and intervention in youth sports. *Behavioral Therapy, 22,* 329–344.
48. Fagone, A. (1991). *Teaching the mental aspects of baseball: A coach's handbook.* Dubuque, IA: William C. Brown Publishers.
49. Sabock, R. (1985). *The coach.* (3rd ed.). Champaign, IL: Human Kinetics Publisher, Inc.
50. Partington, J., & Shangi, G. (1992). Developing and understanding of team psychology. *Int J Sp Psy, 23,* 28–47.
51. Adler, K. (1985). *The art of accompanying and coaching.* Chicago: Dacapo Publishers.
52. Emblen, J. D., & Halstead, L. (1993). Spiritual needs and interventions: Comparing the views of patients, nurses, and chaplains. *Clinical Nurse Specialist, 7,* 175–182.
53. Benner, P. (1985). The oncology clinical use nurse specialist: An expert coach. *Oncology Nursing Forum, 12,* 40–44.
54. Benner, P. (1991). The role of experience, narrative, and community in skilled ethical comportment. *Advances in Nursing Science, 14,* 1–21.
55. Steele, S., & Fenton, M. (1988). Expert practice of clinical nurse specialists. *Clinical Nurse Specialist, 2,* 45–52.
56. McCloskey, J., & Bulechek, G. (1992). *Nursing interventions classification: Taxonomy of nursing interventions.* College of Nursing, The University of Iowa.
57. Lamb, G. S., & Stempel, J. E. (1994). Nurse case management from the client's View: Growing as insider-expert. *Nursing Outlook, 42,* 7–14.
58. Miller, J. (Ed.). (1992). *Coping with chronic illness: Overcoming powerlessness.* (2nd ed.). Philadelphia: F. A. Davis Company.
59. Daloz, L. A. (1986). *Effective teaching and mentoring: Realizing the transformational power of adult learning experiences.* San Francisco: Jossey Bass Publishers.
60. Ferrell, B., Taylor, E., Sattler, G., Fowler, M., & Cheyney, B. (1993). Searching for the meaning of pain: Cancer patients, caregivers, and nurses' perspectives. *Cancer Practice, 1,* 185–194.

Part Four

Humanizing the Experience of Pain and Illness

The Quality of Love

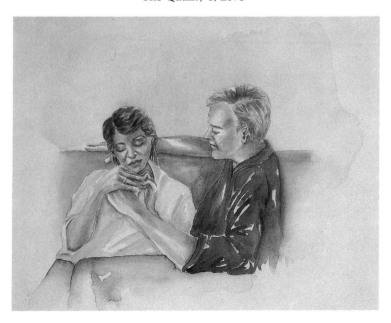

Chapter 9

Humanizing the Experience of Pain and Illness

Betty Rolling Ferrell, PhD, FAAN

City of Hope National Medical Center

The Dehumanization of Pain and Suffering

There is a landmark in the rose garden at the entrance to the City of Hope National Medical Center which we have come to think of as a personal message for our work in quality of life research. The gate reads, "There is no profit in curing the body if in the process we destroy the soul." These few words capture eloquently the challenges facing health-care providers who attempt to minister to those who suffer amidst a system fascinated by technology and cure. There is abundant evidence that advances in health care over recent years have in fact advanced the quantity of life while ignoring issues of quality of life.

Attention to the undertreatment of pain identifies only one aspect of suffering, yet it is representative of our failure to respond to the human experience of life-threatening illnesses such as cancer. While attention to pain is welcome, far less attention has been devoted to the aspect of existential suffering. My intention in editing this book on suffering was to address this neglected aspect of the experience of illness and pain. I was inspired to attempt this project based on those who have influenced my work, including Elisabeth Kubler-Ross (1), Eric Cassel (2), Jeanne Quint Benoliel (3), and other pioneers in the field of palliative care. These leaders have echoed the sentiment that we often care for the tumor, but fail to respond to the person surrounding the tumor.

My interest in issues of high technology pain treatment has been based on the concern that in managing the infusion pump, we often neglect the person attached to the pump. There are many patients for whom suffering will not be remedied by even the strongest of opioid analgesics. Each of the authors in the previous chapters has reflected upon the failures in our health care systems, and society at large, to address the human experiences of illness. Smith concluded his chapter with the admonition that what will help this problem is "not pious talk," but rather moving forward with action to change our approach to patients and their families. These chapters have addressed not only the dehumanization of illness, but also have provided many practical suggestions for humanizing the experiences of patients and family members.

Humanizing Illness and Attention to Suffering

My work, and that of my colleagues, at the City of Hope National Medical Center in the areas of pain and psychosocial needs of cancer patients has been based on a model of quality of life (QOL) as an inclusive concept that incorporates aspects of physical, psychological, social, and spiritual well-being (Figure 9–1). This model has been applied to patients with advanced cancer who are experiencing pain (4), (5), (6), bone marrow transplant (BMT) survivors (7), (8), (9), and, most recently, with long-term survivors of cancer (10) and women with breast cancer (11). In each of our studies, suffering is identified in the domain of spiritual well-being, but in fact, suffering transcends all domains of the model.

FIGURE 9–1   Pain Impacts the Dimensions of Quality of Life

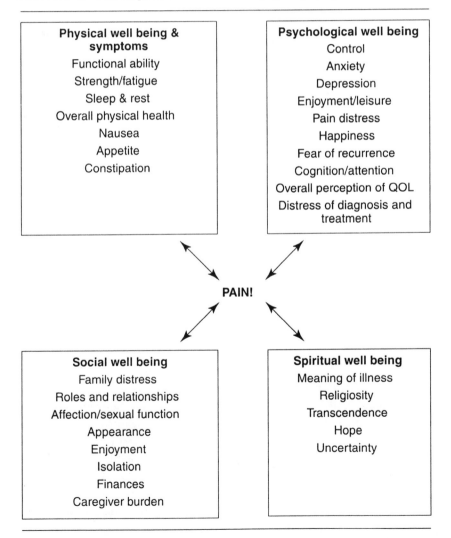

Physical well being & symptoms
Functional ability
Strength/fatigue
Sleep & rest
Overall physical health
Nausea
Appetite
Constipation

Psychological well being
Control
Anxiety
Depression
Enjoyment/leisure
Pain distress
Happiness
Fear of recurrence
Cognition/attention
Overall perception of QOL
Distress of diagnosis and treatment

PAIN!

Social well being
Family distress
Roles and relationships
Affection/sexual function
Appearance
Enjoyment
Isolation
Finances
Caregiver burden

Spiritual well being
Meaning of illness
Religiosity
Transcendence
Hope
Uncertainty

Suffering is not isolated only to those with terminal illness. Rather, it is inherent in the experience of cancer as a life-threatening illness. Across all of our studies, patients and family members have echoed the message that suffering caused by a cancer diagnosis is intensified greatly when healthcare providers fail to respond to psychosocial and spiritual needs. The first and foremost insult rests simply in our failure to listen to the valuable messages of the person facing life-threatening illness, or to believe them. We have heard many stories of the agony that results not only from untreated pain, but also the intensification of the agony when we fail to believe the person's report of pain.

To acknowledge and respect the multidimensional nature of quality of life is to avoid the classic dualism of mind and body separation as described by Cassel (2). It is interesting to note how few measures of quality of life include a spiritual dimension. It is ironic that health care providers often choose to ignore those aspects of quality of life that they are least comfortable with treating, even though these are most critical to the patient.

Patient Suffering

As a staff nurse in an inpatient oncology unit, I recall my early professional experiences in listening to the messages of the terminally ill. As I became more comfortable in conversing with the terminally ill patient, I began to observe the phenomenon of our incompetence in "doing nothing." I recall several instances in which my conversations with patients revealed their decisions to forego further treatment and to inform their physician that they had opted against further chemotherapy. I consistently observed that after the physicians would visit and discuss treatment options, the patients would chose to endure further chemotherapy.

After my first experiences with this phenomenon, I was surprised and confused. How could the patients possibly subject themselves to additional caustic treatments which seemed obviously to lead to further diminished quality of life, separation from family, prolonged hospitalization, and perhaps even hastened morbidity and death? I began to ask patients to explain their decisions to me and I listened intently to their responses. Consistently, I heard patients describe being presented options that they interpreted as a choice of remaining in the hospital surrounded by trusted caregivers when offered even a minuscule chance of hope versus the alternative option of "doing nothing," which they interpreted often as abandonment. Unfortunately, the absence of aggressive, curative treatment too often resembles "doing nothing." Those committed to palliative care would suggest that this alternative treatment should also be aggressive and one of hope, albeit in a different form.

The past decade has focused largely on one aspect of advanced disease, the undertreatment of patients in the area of pain management. A decade of literature has questioned how it is that an advanced, highly technological healthcare system could possibly fail to respond to patients in pain. The data regarding our attention to pain as a symptom is almost astonishing. How is it that medical students receive only one or two hours of content focused on pain? How is it that major cancer centers, caring for patients whom are expected to experience moderate to severe pain, can fail to have even basic pain assessment procedures in place or fail to provide specialty services such as palliative care programs?

Perhaps in many ways, we have focused on the microscopic issue of pain, although critically important, while failing to acknowledge the larger overriding issue related to this problem. The undertreatment of pain is in fact symptomatic of the overall attention given to the dying patient in this country. Over the past two decades, much has been written to speculate on the cause of the undertreatment of pain, yet the answer likely rests within the reality that we have done such a poor job of caring for the dying.

Pain, throughout our research, is viewed as a metaphor for death by both patients and family caregivers (12), (13). To deny the presence of pain is one further means of denying impending death. The challenge reflected in the preceding chapters is to make palliative care more than "doing nothing." It is essential that palliative care is also aggressive care. As Shapiro explained, doing a physical exam on a patient for whom no additional diagnostic findings are expected is still a means of demonstrating continued concern, a continued relationship rather than abandonment, and as a form of touch.

Another critical concept cited in this text is that of control. This concept has also been evident throughout our research in areas of pain and quality of life. In one study we conducted to validate the concept of quality of life for patients in pain, two concepts emerged as being critically important to patients and yet were absent in our measures of quality of life (5). The first of these concepts was that of control. Patients explained that being in pain made them feel out of control. While cancer, AIDS, or other life-threatening illnesses may have had a devastating effect on the person's life, it is often the presence of pain that signals a loss of control and independence. Interventions that enhance a patient's sense of control are profound influences on the patient's quality of life. I am reminded of a patient in one of our first studies in bone marrow transplant and QOL. This woman described how during her prolonged course of hospitalization in the bone marrow transplant unit she became quite obsessed with her bedside table. She spent hours each day rearranging the few personal possessions on the bedside table. She became outraged when a member of the staff would lay medical supplies on it or touch her belongings, to the point that the staff believed her behavior was a sign of isolation psychosis.

In retrospect, the patient explained that during her course of illness, she felt her life had become unwound as she had day-by-day given up another layer of control. Upon hospitalization she had lost control of her future, knowing full well the high morbidity associated with BMT. Isolated from her family, she lost control of any interaction with her children and the decisions in her home. As her condition worsened, she lost control of even the most basic of physical functions and personal care. The woman came to realize that the bedside table was the only thing over which she had control and struggled desperately to maintain it. This story is a poignant reminder of the intricacies in our care which serve either to intensify or diminish the suffering associated with an illness experience.

The experience of suffering for patients is one intertwined with the meaning of illness and pain. Persons living with cancer often find meaning by construing benefit from their illness (14), (15), (16). Outcomes of life reappraisal include an increased appreciation for human relationships, greater self-understanding, and stronger positive attitudes regarding life. Patients with cancer also find meaning for their illness by reliance on beliefs in fate or probability, and appealing to a higher order or faith (17), (18).

Patient suffering extends beyond physical symptoms to the impact of illness on social and psychological well-being. As a woman with breast cancer described, ". . . when I look in the mirror, the person that looks back at me is not somebody I like the looks of" (11). The altered appearance resulting from a devastating illness is a major threat to the intactness of the person, described by Cassel as suffering (2). The suffering associated with AIDS, as described in the chapter by Saunders, is undoubtedly intensified by the extreme devastation of the physical body associated with that disease.

Our research has also revealed the intensified suffering apparent when patients perceive their illness was avoidable or that their diagnosis was delayed. Another woman with breast cancer expressed her suffering in saying her illness was a ". . . very traumatic thing, having been misdiagnosed because I essentially walked around with the tumor for a year and a half. So that's the hard part of this disease is that what "I'm going through now, somebody did this to me (11)."

Our studies have also demonstrated the aloneness of living with life-threatening illness. Suffering is diminished when healthcare providers take the time to refer patients to support groups so that they receive the sustenance provided only by a shared community of suffering.

Family Suffering

In our program of research related to pain and quality of life we have had the opportunity to interview many family members to gain their perspective of cancer and pain. Our interviews generally begin with an open question such as, "Tell me what it has been like for you, having someone you love with cancer." Often, the answer comes first in the form of tears and a common expression of, "Thank God, someone finally asked."

Family members have shared their experiences of being frequent visitors in hospitals and clinics, often over years of treatments, yet never once being acknowledged or asked about their experience as a family caregiver also experiencing the illness. When family members have been asked to describe the patient's pain, their descriptions have included terms such as "agonizing, excruciating, horrible, inconceivable, miserable, overwhelming, terrible, unbearable, and uncontrollable"—clearly expressions of the suffering felt by observers of pain (12), (13).

Family members have described physical sensations of observing their loved one's in pain. As one husband described, "She's hurting, and it makes me cry. It's like a knife twisting in her." Another spouse described the pain as "a burning sensation like a branding iron. Within the last month, she has been in agonizing pain, with wild eyes. She felt like she was being stabbed with a knife. She felt like her insides were blowing up" (12).

We have observed that the family experience of pain is one of helplessness. Many husbands described cancer pain much like watching their wives in labor—observing intense physical pain yet feeling that there was little they could do. Our research has also revealed that this sense of helplessness is greatly reduced when family members become involved in aggressive care for the patient's pain, such as involvement in medications and nondrug pain treatments (13).

Family suffering is an experience intertwined within the relationship between patient and the individual family member. Observing one's child in pain is distinct from caring for a spouse after 50 years of marriage or from the experience of watching an elderly parent in pain. Caring for an elderly parent in pain will often entail a reversal of roles, or feelings of failure as the family caregiver isn't able to return the care they have received from the parent.

A stark reality is that the last hours of a patient's life are in fact the memories the family will hold forever. Failing to respond to a child dying in unrelieved pain creates momentary agony for the child, but an eternal memory for the parents. Similarly, providing optimum comfort during the final hours of a life creates a memory of comfort and diminishes the suffering associated with the loss of a loved one (19), (20).

Attention to family suffering, much like tending to the patient, begins by listening and believing (19). A mother expressed the comfort of being referred to a pain service in saying, "It was important to us even to have a group of people that believed him because that can make you sick too, thinking—I feel it and everybody says that it's not real—and, it turned out to be darn real at the end when it had already done all of it's damage" (20).

Caring for a loved one in pain is often described by family members as an existential crisis in which they seek to find support from God to endure the experience, while at the same time blaming God for causing the illness and pain. A parent described this struggle in saying, "I can't hide that. I ask Him a hundred times, 'Why are You doing this with my son?' An innocent child . . . why do you have to put him through this pain? If You want him, just take him, and don't make him suffer like this." I ask God that question a lot of times" (19).

Many families have also expressed that the initial diagnosis of cancer in fact brought the family closer together. However, as the illness continued and pain dominated, the families were often destroyed. A parent caring for a child in pain said, "We were as a family, but I was pushed pretty far by the pain . . . the day he went in where he was screaming, and the nurse came and gave him the pain machine—Henry sat down and said, 'It's over. I can't, I don't want to live another day. I can't live another day seeing him like this.' I sat down, and I was crying. Pete was crying. Everybody was crying. See, we had a good family; but, how much can you watch? How much suffering can you watch from your child, your 7-year-old child, and still keep your mind? So I would say, we were a close family; but I'll tell you, cancer can kill a close family" (19).

Throughout our studies we have attempted to distinguish the devasting experience of a illness, such as cancer, from the effects of pain. A mother very eloquently captured this in saying that having a child diagnosed with cancer was like "watching your child dangled over a river." She then described the difference in stating that having the child in pain was like "watching your child dropped into a river and drown." The message for healthcare providers is that in fact we must watch many family members whose lives are dangled over a river—yet, we do not need to force them to fall into a river and drown. Attention to the needs of the terminally ill can in fact reduce the unnecessary suffering of terminal illness.

Conclusion

The dehumanization of illness is avoidable; there is in fact much we can do to humanize the experiences of illness and even the moment of death. Suffering, as Kahn and Steeves have described, is exhaustion of the spirit. Attention to the spiritual needs of the patient is a crucial step toward alleviation of suffering.

Dunlop reminds us that we must recognize that our challenge begins with altering the education provided to healthcare professionals, particularly within medical schools. People cannot practice what they do not know, and will not know what we do not teach. As Smith described in his chapter on the theological perspective of suffering, we must integrate lessons of compassion and empathy to improve our care of patients in pain.

Wisdom regarding the recognition and alleviation of suffering can be found in great literary and scientific works by leaders in the field of palliative care. One of the most important messages I have read came though from an editorial, "On Deeper Reflection," written by a medical student. In this editorial, Dr. Greg Sachs described his experience as a resident while admitting an 87-year-old woman to a geriatric unit.

The woman had multiple problems including dementia, incontinence, diabetes, pressure sores, and malnutrition. The woman screamed in pain as Dr. Sachs examined a large pressure sore over her right trochanter. He saw movement in the wound, and initially feared there might be maggots present. On deeper reflection, he realized that the movement paralled his own motion and that in fact he was seeing his own reflection on the shiny surface of her hip prosthesis. Dr. Sachs synthesized this experience in writing:

> Seeing oneself in a pressure sore is a stark and frightening vision, disturbing on many levels. In addition to the grotesque wound and personal reflection, it seemed to mirror the topsy-turvy medical care given to many such patients. Mrs. Smith came from a hospital where she received mechanical ventilation for a respiratory arrest suffered when she was hypoglycemic. She had pleural effusions tapped and analyzed and innumerable laboratory tests performed. Yet she lay long enough without being turned for all the tissue between her skin and bones to necrotize.
>
> It is sad that somewhere in the course of a dementing process Mrs. Smith lost many of the characteristics that most of us associate with meaningful adult human life. It is sadder still that she received medical treatment that forgot about her as a human being (22).

Much like this experience, our failure to respond to pain and suffering is no less than a moral outrage. Those who care for persons with cancer and other life-threatening illnesses face erosion of the human spirit no less destructive than a decubitus ulcer, yet perhaps less visible. On deeper reflection into the eyes of our patients and their families, we too can humanize systems of care and diminish the experience of suffering.

References

1. Kubler Ross, E. (1969). *On death and dying.* New York: MacMillan.
2. Cassel, E. (1982). The nature of suffering and the goal of medicine. *New England Journal of Medicine, 306,* 639–645.
3. Quint, J. (1967). *The nurse and the dying patient.* New York: MacMillan.
4. Ferrell, B. R., Wisdom, C., Wenzl, C., & Schneider, C. (1989). Quality of life as an outcome variable in pain research. *Cancer, 63,* 2321–2327.
5. Padilla, G., Ferrell, B. R., Grant, M., & Rhiner, M. (1990). Defining the content domain of quality of life for cancer patients with pain. *Cancer Nursing, 13,* 108–115.

6. Ferrell, B. R., Grant, M., Padilla, G., & Rhiner, M. (1991). Patient perceptions of pain and quality of life. *The Hospice Journal, 7,* 9–24.
7. Grant, M., Ferrell, B. R., Schmidt, G. M., Fonbuena, P., Niland, J. C., & Forman, S. J. (1992). Measurement of quality of life in bone marrow transplantation survivors. *Quality of Life Research, 1,* 375–384.
8. Ferrell, B., Grant, M., Schmidt, G. M., Rhiner, M., Whitehead, C., Fonbuena, P., & Forman, S. J. (1992). The meaning of quality of life for bone marrow transplant survivors. Part 1: The impact of bone marrow transplant on quality of life. *Cancer Nursing, 15,* 153–160.
9. Ferrell, B., Grant, M., Schmidt, G. M., Rhiner, M., Whitehead, C., & Fonbuena, P. (1992). The meaning of quality of life for bone marrow transplant survivors. Part 2: Improving quality of life for bone marrow transplant survivors. *Cancer Nursing, 15,* 247–253.
10. Ferrell, B. R., Hassey-Dow, K., & Leigh, S. (in press). Quality of life in cancer survivors. *Breast Cancer Treatment and Research.*
11. Ferrell, B., Grant, M., Garcia, N., Otis-Green, S., & Funk, B. (1995). Pain and quality of life in breast cancer. Research in progress.
12. Ferrell, B. R., Rhiner, M., Cohen, M., & Grant, M. (1991). Pain as a metaphor for illness. Part I: Impact of cancer pain on family caregivers. *Oncology Nursing Forum, 18,* 1303–1309.
13. Ferrell, B. R., Cohen, M., Rhiner, M., & Rozek, A. (1991). Pain as a metaphor for illness. Part II: Family caregivers' management of pain. *Oncology Nursing Forum, 18,* 1315–1321.
14. Taylor, S. E. (1983). Adjustment to threatening events: A theory of cognitive adaptation. *American Psychology, 38,* 1161–1173.
15. Johnston, E. (1992). *The search for meaning among persons living with recurrent cancer.* Unpublished doctoral dissertation, University of Pennsylvania, Philadelphia.
16. Haberman, M. R. (1987). *Living with leukemia: The personal meaning attributed to illness and treatment by Adults undergoing a bone marrow transplantation.* Unpublished doctoral dissertation, University of Washington.
17. Steeves, R. H. (1988). *The experience of suffering and meaning in bone marrow transplant patients.* Unpublished doctoral dissertation, University of Washington.
18. Ferrell, B. R., Johnston, T. E., Sattler, G., Fowler, M., & Cheyney, L. (1993). Searching for the meaning of pain: Cancer patients', caregivers', and nurses' perspectives. *Cancer Practice, 1,* 185–194.
19. Ferrell, B. R., Rhiner, M., Shapiro, B., & Dierkes, M. (1994). The experience of pediatric cancer pain. Part I: Impact of pain on the family. *Journal of Pediatric Nursing, 9,* 368–379.
20. Rhiner, M., Ferrell, B. R., Shapiro, B., & Dierkes, M. (1994). The experience of pediatric cancer pain. Part II: Management of pain. *Journal of Pediatric Nursing, 9,* 380–387.
21. Ferrell, B. R., Rhiner, M., Shapiro, B., & Strause, L. (1994). The family experience of cancer pain management in children. *Cancer Practice, 2,* 441–446.
22. Sachs, G. (1988). On deeper reflection. *JAMA, 259,* 2145.

Index